W9-DHM-505

About the author

Chris Beyrer teaches at the School of Hygiene and Public Health at Johns Hopkins University, Baltimore, USA. An epidemiologist, he has worked and travelled extensively in South East Asia.

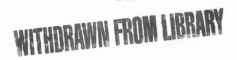

WITHDRAWN FROM LIBRARY

For Henry Peter Lange and
for Faith Doherty

WITHDRAWN FROM LIBRARY

MONTGOMERY COLLEGE
ROCKVILLE CAMPUS LIBRARY
ROCKVILLE, MARYLAND

WAR IN THE BLOOD
Sex, politics and AIDS in Southeast Asia

Chris Beyrer

White Lotus
BANGKOK

Zed Books Ltd
LONDON & NEW YORK

289940

JUL 2 6 2004

War in the Blood was first published by Zed Books Ltd,
7 Cynthia Street, London N1 9JF, UK, and Room 400,
175 Fifth Avenue, New York, NY 10010, USA, in 1998.

Published in Burma, Cambodia, Laos and Thailand by
White Lotus Company Ltd, GPO Box 1141, Bangkok
10501, Thailand, in 1998.

Copyright © Chris Beyrer, 1998.

Cover designed by Andrew Corbett
Set in Monotype Baskerville and Univers by Ewan Smith
Printed and bound in the United Kingdom
by Biddles Ltd, Guildford and King's Lynn

The right of Chris Beyrer to be identified as the author of this work has
been asserted by him in accordance with the Copyright, Designs and
Patents Act, 1988.

Distributed exclusively in the United States by St Martin's Press, Inc.,
175 Fifth Avenue, New York, NY 10010, USA.

A catalogue record for this book is available from the British Library.

Cataloging-in-publication data has been applied for from the Library
of Congress.

ISBN 1 85649 531 0 cased
ISBN 1 85649 532 9 limp

In Burma, Cambodia, Laos and Thailand
ISBN 974 8434 31 1 limp

Contents

Preface

The book you have in your hands is something of an experiment. It has grown out of several of years of work, at times exhilarating and at times deeply frustrating, on one problem: the swift and pervasive spread of the HIV virus among the people of mainland Southeast Asia. It is not intended to be an academic text in my field – public health – though much of the information included is the result of research in public health, epidemiology, and prevention. What I've tried to do is exploratory, provisional, and personal. The result is as much, at times, a travel book as a medical one. A journey on the AIDS road, and one by no means complete.

This road led to seven countries: Thailand, Burma, Malaysia, Cambodia, Vietnam, Laos, and China. These states include emerging democracies, a military dictatorship, three of the world's five remaining Communist regimes, and an Islamic Republic. They include four of the most rapidly growing economies and three of the poorest nations on earth. The contrasts and the diversity of Southeast Asia today are striking and daunting; if you looked at forest policy or family planning programs, the state of civil society or of human rights, you'd undoubtedly find differences as marked as those revealed in these seven countries' responses to AIDS. But because HIV spread involves sex, and drug use, and the state of health care, looking at how countries as different and Burma and Malaysia have responded can tell us a great deal about life in these places. About life at its seediest and most criminal, and people at their most inspiring and courageous.

The choice of countries discussed here may seem eccentric, and to require some explanation. The region's most important political grouping is ASEAN, the Association of Southeast Asian Nations. It now includes seven member states: Brunei, Indonesia, Malaysia, the Philippines, Singapore, Thailand and Vietnam. Cambodia, Laos, and

vii

Burma have observer status, and are expected to become full members by the year 2000. I have not attempted to include all the ASEAN member states here. The archipelagic nations of Indonesia and the Philippines are not addressed for several reasons, most importantly because they are not countries I felt I understood well enough to discuss them, despite their clear regional importance. The city states of Brunei and Singapore have also been excluded, again partly because I know them little, but also because Singapore has not consistently reported HIV statistics to international bodies. I have included China because the evidence suggests that AIDS in Yunnan, to date China's most HIV-affected Province, is tightly linked to Southeast Asia, to Burma and the Golden Triangle heroin industry. While India is not formally presented here, and is certainly not a part of Southeast Asia, I have discussed some aspects of the Indian situation throughout the text, as the burgeoning Indian HIV epidemic appears to be following the early Thai pattern closely, at least as far as very rapid heterosexual spread is concerned. If HIV spreads in India for a few more years at current rates, the majority of Asians with HIV will be Indians; lessons learned in smaller countries may be sorely needed there.

I have tried to portray the people and places on the AIDS road with as much honesty as possible, but in the case of several countries, I have deliberately had to change or omit names, places, and information sources. I have endeavored to confirm independently what was said and have not altered the information given. I have lived and worked in Thailand, visited and taught in Malaysia and China as an official guest, and have traveled and researched in several other countries without permission – in the case of Burma, sometimes without visa or passport. Several governments explicitly criticized here have not had the chance to respond. But in some countries choices have to be made; it is difficult to meet both dissidents and officials. When such a choice had to be made, I went with the people, not their leaders, which perhaps both weakens and strengthens what is written here.

I have taken considerable license in going well beyond the boundaries of my field, public health, in this attempt. Beyond hubris, the only explanation I can offer is that this disease has called on all concerned to use the tools of disciplines as diverse as history, anthropology, virology, and political science to seek solutions. In all these fields I am a rank amateur. Professionals will immediately see the shortcomings of this approach, the perhaps unavoidable fate of a generalist's attempt in fields rich with impressive specialists. Though epidemiology is in part a quantitative science, I have tried to keep the math as simple as possible; there is little beyond percentage points, and some simple rates. Again, specialists may find this frustrating. More detailed information and the scientific sources from which it has been derived is included in the notes and references.

If my arguments seem heated, and the rhetoric less than dispassionate, the responsibility is mine. So too are responsibilities to friends living with HIV/AIDS, and to friends, lovers, and colleagues already gone – people whose integrity shames any attempt to mask what one thinks, knows or feels. AIDS began its killing onslaught in New York while I was a medical student; it has always been a part of my work in medicine, and it has been a source of deep personal pain. I lived for seven years in what epidemiologists call a 'discordant couple': one of us infected, the other not. My partner died in my arms in 1991. Shortly thereafter I moved to northern Thailand, just in time to see another city, Chiang Mai, fall into the withering embrace of mine enemy. It is my ardent belief that the HIV disasters which befell New York City and Chiang Mai need not be repeated. Watching them being repeated has driven the text you have in your hands. The extent to which this experiment is of use to others involved in similar struggles is the measure of its success.

This book could not have been written without the assistance and courage of many people who cannot be named. My debts to them all are deep, as is my respect for the risks they took in speaking frankly.

In Thailand I would like to thank Dr Chirasak Khamboonruang for his constant support, Dr Chawalit Natpratan and his staff, Khun Piyada Kunawararak, Dr Sakol Eiumtrakul of Kawila Army Hospital, Mrs Somboon Suprasert of the Thai Red Cross, Dr Tippawan Prapamontol, Dr Sodsai Tovanbutra, Dr Sungwal Rugpao, Acharn Wanpen Eamjoy and the staff at the Research Institute for Health Sciences, Chiang Mai University. Friends and colleagues who provided invaluable information and conversation include Dr Henry Stephens, Jackie Pollock, Dr Kate Bond, Prof. Chayan Vaddhanaphuti, Bertil Lintner, Gordon Fairclough, Dr Pasakorn Akarasewi, Sally Thompson, and Jan Willem der Lind Van Wijngaarden and the staff of

Chaai Chuay Chaai. Burmese friends and colleagues have been
invaluable sources of information and encouragement. I would like
to thank Dr Naing Aung, Dr Thaung Htun, and Aung Myo Myint of
the All-Burma Students Democratic Front, Harn Yawnghwe of the
Burma Donors Secretariat, Dr Myint Cho, Mr Michael Jalla of the
Pan-Kachin Development Society, Dr Sann Aung of the National
Coalition Government of the Union of Burma, and Ko Zaw Gyi. Ko
Tint Aung and Ma San San Myint shared their family and their
stories. The Burmese Federation of Trade Unions provided some
important data; their courage has been remarkable. To those inside
Burma, my thanks and my prayers. In Malaysia I would like to
acknowledge the Malaysian AIDS Council, the people of Pink
Triangle, and the invaluable assistance of Hisham Hussein, Palani
Narayaran, and Khartini Salmah. At the University of Malaya my
colleagues Dr Ng Kee Peng, Dr Ken Lam, and Prof. Y. Ngeow all
provided insight and understanding. For introducing me to the Ven.
Maha Ghosananda, deep thanks to Yeshua Mosher. To Maha himself,
I can only acknowledge an unpayable debt. The staff of the
Cambodian Women's Development Association welcomed me with
kindness. Invaluable assistance was provided by Ms Chantal Oung.
Nina Reznick was an essential partner on the road. The staff of
Médecins Sans Frontières and of the International Red Cross helped
to fathom the situation in rural Cambodia. Dr Xiao-Fang Yu of
Johns Hopkins University, Dr Ximing Chao, Dr Rosalyn Fon, and
individuals from the Kachin and Wa nationality were of real assistance in China. Friends and colleagues in Laos and Vietnam were
candid and brave; I hope to be able to acknowledge them by name in
the future. My colleagues at Johns Hopkins University gave both
support and freedom, for I which I thank particularly Dr Ken Nelson
and Prof. David Celentano. Thanks also to Dr Jean Carr, Dr Andrew
Artenstein, and Dr John McNeil, colleagues at Walter Reed whose
work informs much of this text. Minka Nyhuis gave two precious
gifts – her friendship and a quiet place to write.

Part One
Countries

1. Introduction

In mid-July 1996, an estimated 21.8 million adults and children worldwide were living with HIV/AIDS, of whom 20.4 million (94 percent) were in the developing world. Close to 19 million adults and children (86 percent of the world total) were living with HIV/AIDS in sub-Saharan Africa, and in South and Southeast Asia. Of the adults, 12.2 million (58 percent) were male and 8.8 million (42 percent) were female.

Worldwide during 1995, 2.7 million new adult HIV infections occurred (averaging more that 7,000 new infections each day). Of these, about 1 million (an average of nearly 3,000 new infections per day) occurred in Southeast Asia, and 1.4 million were in sub-Saharan Africa. The industrialized world accounted for about 55,000 new HIV infections in 1995 (nearly 150 new infections per day: about 2 percent of the global total).

In 1995 approximately 500,000 children were born with HIV infection (about 1,400 per day); of these children 67 percent were in sub-Saharan Africa, 30 percent in South and Southeast Asia, and 2 to 3 percent in Latin America and the Caribbean.

Since the beginning of the pandemic, 26 million HIV infections (93 percent of the total) have occurred in the developing world. The number of HIV-infected people in South and Southeast Asia is now more than twice the total number of infected people in the entire industrialized world.

UNAIDS. The Status and Trends of the Global HIV/AIDS Pandemic, July 1996

Highway 107 runs due north from Chiang Mai, Thailand's second largest city, and for 700 years the gateway to the fabled Golden Triangle, to Fang, a trading town just short of the northern border with Burma. Chiang Mai is circled by a ring road which peels off several highways, including 107. Driving along the stretch inside the ring road, lined with shopping malls and discount outlets, truck depots and shiny new gas stations, it's easy to agree with the Thais that their modern kingdom can hardly be called 'developing' or 'Third World': the ring around the old city is as thoroughly developed as it is unattractive. Stuck with you in the ubiquitous traffic are a seemingly

3

impossible number of late model cars – Mercedes Benz's, BMWs, Mitsubishi Land Rovers, Pajero jeeps. A decade of double-digit annual economic growth has generated real, if unevenly distributed, wealth. Once you take the turn north, the communities that support both the shopping arcades and the first-class traffic begin to appear. Suburban Chiang Mai was once mostly fruit orchards and paddy fields, scattered farming communities and country *wats* (temples). Much of it was forest. You can still see some fruit trees, even the occasional paddy, but what predominates are sprawling housing developments, condominium sub-divisions, and golf courses. Take away the transplanted palms and the odd Thai touch to a roof gable, and you could be heading north out of Fort Lauderdale or Atlanta. The old-style Thai houses that remain along the road, their dark teak frames beaten down by monsoons and the potent northern sun, look fragile and transitory scattered among the developments, like memories already half-forgotten.

As you leave Chiang Mai behind, heading north out of the valley of the Ping River, the balance between new and old, rich and poor, starts to shift. After about 60 kilometers the condos cease, cattle appear, and water buffaloes, fields of bean and garlic. Houses are more and more of wood, less prosperous, fewer. Soon after you come to Chiang Dao, Mountain of Stars, a single limestone crag that announces the coming climb. The mountains here are not high, the peaks are all under 5,000 feet, but they are densely packed and steep, the eastern-most tail of the Himalayas. The forest cover is secondary or tertiary, the teak stands are a memory, like the elephant herds that foraged here till the 1930s. The town of Chiang Dao, nestled in these crags, is easy to miss; the major employer is an army camp, and the service sector around it, which includes a half-dozen or so cheap brothels, some beer halls, a video parlor.

From here to Fang it's another 200 kilometers of mountains falling to hills, narrow valleys cut by the Ping, occasional villages. The traffic is long gone; people up here are on motorcycles, or packed to standing in the back of pick-ups. Many are not Thai. You find Hmong, Lisu, Lahu, and Akha tribespeople in these districts. The men dressed like Thai farmers, the women a rainbow of richly colored cloths, elaborate headdresses, the babies they carry bundles bright as birds.

Coming into Fang after the drive is something of a disappointment. The town, a smallish farming and trading post, simply starts, without any obvious relation to the hills behind it. Most of the buildings are concrete block shophouses built along either side of Highway 107. There's a bus station, a truck depot, a disproportionate number of banks. The Burmese border is still 25 kilometers further north. The place has little to offer the tourist or traveler – most pass right through it heading for Thaton, where the twisty Kok River comes out of Burma and runs east to Chiang Rai, on the base of the Golden Triangle. Boat trips on the Kok are popular, the scenery lovely; paddy fields and banana groves along the shore give way to rolling green foothills, and they to bluish mountains in the distance.

The first time I went to Fang, shortly after moving to Thailand in 1992, I went with two nurses from the Thai Ministry of Public Health and a professor from Chiang Mai University. Fang was going to be one of our study sites for a research project on HIV, the virus that causes AIDS.[1] Though Fang is about as far from bustling Bangkok, the Thai capital, as you can go and still be in Thailand, the district had already reported astonishingly high rates of HIV infection among its farmers and traders. The 25-bed district hospital was fast becoming an AIDS care centre; close to half the admissions were for HIV-related illnesses. Despite its seeming isolation, and the lazy rural air of Fang's dozen or so dusty streets, the community was going to be as hard hit as San Francisco or Kinshasa.

We were met in the hospital parking lot by the Director, a smiling man in his late thirties named Dr Samadjarn, thankfully fluent in English. He and seven nurses were clinical staff of the hospital. We sat down to tea and pleasantries, introductions were made all around, and friends and colleagues asked after. The atmosphere, new to me then and ever after a delight, was warm, polite but engaging, calm yet energized, more like a reunion of old friends than a medical meeting. The Fang staff were eager to be part of our project. It was soon clear to us all that they could do what we were asking. That they wanted to know more, to do more. It was also clear that the staff from Chiang Mai and from Fang had already agreed to the collaboration – the visit was a formality, but an essential one; we had to know each other and we had to visit their district if we were going to work together. The hard parts – negotiations, budgets, staff assignments – had been worked out well in advance of our trip.

When the meeting was over, we toured the facilities. The inpatient

ward was full; it would always be so when we returned. There were
three patients getting intravenous drips of amphotericin B, an anti-
fungal drug used in AIDS: two men and a woman, all farmers, and
all with the same disease, *penicillosis* – a blood, multi-organ and skin
infection caused by a fungus of extreme rarity outside this region,
but common among people with AIDS in these hills. (It causes
unmistakable black-centered lesions on the skin; untreated, it is
uniformly fatal.) The hospital had a basic lab, two private counseling
rooms, an STD (sexually transmitted disease) clinic, an x-ray
machine. Everything was fairly simple but clean and functioning.
The outpatient service had an open-air waiting room with several
rows of long wooden benches under a fiberglass roof. We were a
welcome distraction from the wait – a white face was clearly novel –
much pointing and giggling went on, children hiding behind their
mothers, bubbles of talk. They seemed to be poor, rural people, like
their neighbors with AIDS on the ward, Thais and a mix of Tribal
minorities in their distinctive costumes. The nurses called them *Chao
Kow*, people of the mountains.

In the afternoon we were taken on a tour of the district. Dr
Samadjarn was not from Fang; he'd been assigned to the hospital by
the Government, but he'd come to know the area well. We drove out
of town and into the low hills off to the west, toward Burma.
Scattered villages, fields, orchards of mango and litchi, small herds
of thin, long-eared Brahma cattle. The road followed a branch of
the Kok higher into the hills. We turned off it quite suddenly and
veered steeply down into a wide, shallow valley. A manicured valley
of orange trees, row upon row of them, filling the floor right to its
steep walls and rolling back up it almost out of sight. In the distance,
beyond the groves, was a cement dam. Above it, a large reservoir
had been built to hold water for the trees. 'The second largest citrus
orchard in Southeast Asia,' said Dr Samadjarn, with some pride.
The orchard (and its dam and processing plant) was a foreign-funded
development project making orange-juice concentrate for export.
There were a good many workers among the rows, men and women
in wide straw hats and huge floppy rubber boots – spraying in-
secticide out of metal drums strapped on their backs. It looked like
hot work.

We stopped for sodas in the home of the owner, a large structure
of gleaming golden teak, built in the old Thai style but clearly very

new. Then Dr Samadjarn suggested we visit a nearby village. There was a family there he needed to visit, and whom he wanted us to meet. Their village, about five kilometers downriver from the orchard, was also new, but it wasn't built in any style – cheap tin roofed shacks, several little palm-thatched shops selling cigarettes, soap, whiskey, a few low concrete houses, and, unusually for a Thai village, no *wat*. The place, we learned, was actually the result of the relocation of three older villages. These had been drowned out when the dam went up, and the villagers moved here.

We parked our van in some shade near the road and walked through the village on a dirt track, dry and hard in this season. There were few people moving. Most of the able-bodied were away, working in the orchard or farther afield. In the front yards of the houses, tending small gardens or sitting in shade, were some older people and young children. On the far end of the settlement, almost to the hills at its back, we stopped at a small house hidden behind some tangled vines. An elderly couple were sitting on plastic mats spread on the ground beside the house, a ramshackle structure which looked completely dark inside. The woman smiled warmly and *wai*-ed[2] Dr Samadjarn as we approached. They spoke for a few moments, the old lady puffing away on a thick, pungent cigar. The old man seemed lost in a dream, and never looked our way. I noticed a boy of about eight or nine, very thin and dark, carrying a baby in his arms. He was standing about 20 feet behind the old people, peering from beside a tree. When I smiled at him he moved carefully off towards the house, dropping the baby with the old lady on his way. They were all in rags; the boy in just a pair of stained, ashy shorts, the baby naked, the old lady in a faded sarong, the old man in a pair of green fatigue trousers black with grime, his gaunt chest laced with tattoos. A few minutes later a man of about 30 appeared, in a tee-shirt and gym shorts, stumbling out of the house into the sharp sunlight. He looked thin, though handsome, a larger version of his son. His eyes, when he stood closer, were yellow and watery.

The man, the father of the two boys and the son of the old couple, greeted Dr Samadjarn with obvious pleasure and warmth. He shouted to the boy who ran off and came back with a teapot full of water and some glasses. We drank the water standing, while Dr Samadjarn and the young man spoke at length. One of the nurses picked up the baby, who flopped in her arms half-asleep. The baby looked pale against her skin, his proportions not right: head too large, limbs too thin, belly tense. Dr Samadjarn handed the man a white paper bag, and spoke to me in English, which he assured me none of them understood.

'This man was one of my first AIDS patients. Clinically he is doing fairly well, but now he has some depression. His wife died three weeks ago. This is the first time I've seen him since the cremation. The baby is also positive, I wanted to make sure he brought him to see us in the next few days. The older boy is alright; he was born, I think, before the problem started. I'm not sure the old people really understand what will happen. They are very simple people. The grandfather has senility, too, what you call Alzheimers in America. The older boy is the biggest problem; he is very intelligent and seems to understand what's going on. His father just told me he stopped talking some days ago.'

The father followed us out to the van where the nurses gave him a big bag of oranges from the orchard. He *wai*-ed them deeply, then me, then Dr Samadjarn. He stood waiting by the roadside as we drove off, not moving, just holding the oranges above the dust.

On the long, hot drive back to Chiang Mai I feigned sleep. The site visit had gone well; Fang looked like a good place for our project. But I could not get the older boy out of my mind: his dark eyes, his silence. He had just lost his mother, and he was going to lose his father and his brother. The family was already poor, and going to get poorer fast.

I had been struck by several things on this, my first home visit to a Thai family dealing with AIDS: by the curiously warm yet formal relationship of the father and Dr Samadjarn; by the poverty of the family and their community, so striking after Chiang Mai; by the massive orange grove outside Fang; by the squalor of the new settlement (Dr Samadjarn told me after we'd left that the village, which had perhaps 1,800 inhabitants, had two competing brothels and a shooting gallery for heroin users); most of all by the face of AIDS in this place, so different from what I'd known in Baltimore and New York, where I'd worked (and lived) in another AIDS crisis. No matter how much one reads, it takes time and exposure to realize the implications of saying, 'In developing countries the majority of cases of HIV infection are due to heterosexual transmission.' The difference was in the face of a young father knowing he would not survive to provide for his children, in the eyes of an old lady about to have her world destroyed. Most of all in the mute pain of a boy whose prospects were declining as sharply as his father's resistance to disease.

I've been back to Fang many times since that first visit. Our project there did go very well, so well in fact that we didn't identify any incident[3] infections. By 1995 Fang Hospital had a truly impressive integrated AIDS care program, with a visiting nurse service, even a full-time social worker to deal with job loss and AIDS discrimination. But I've also come to know other sides of Fang, darker and more difficult realities without which it would be impossible to understand why the district's communities have been so hard hit.

In 1994 colleagues of mine began an HIV prevention project in the brothels of Chiang Mai, Chiang Dao, and Mae Rim, a Chiang Mai suburb. About half of the women they met working in these sex venues were from Burma. My colleagues, social scientists, began with some simple questions: Where are you from? How did you get here? The women's stories quickly began to be repeated: virtually all the women had come via just three routes. Fang was a central stop on the largest of these. It was a center for the trafficking of women and girls from Burma to the brothels of Thailand. The women had other stories to tell; Fang was where newly trafficked women were 'broken in' to the sex industry. It will probably never be known how many women (it's in the thousands) have been repeatedly raped and brutalized there before the transport south. Highway 107 carries them to the army camp at Chiang Dao, and further south, to Chiang Mai, Bangkok, and from there to Tokyo.

Many of the people working in the district's orchards are Burmese as well, ethnic refugees and migrant laborers from the civil war raging just over the green hills to the west. They work for a pittance and have no more rights than the women in the brothels. Like them, they are subject to constant harassment from the authorities, and pay out a fair proportion of their wages in bribes to avoid repatriation. Fear of the authorities keeps the migrant workers away from health care, from HIV information, from safety. Some of the other workers are Thai farmers who have lost their land to the dam project or others like it, and many have yet to be compensated. This is what happened to the family I met on that first visit. After they'd lost their land, the wife had gone to work in Bangkok in order to feed the family. Like many northern women with low education and no work experience beyond field and market, she'd drifted into the sex trade. (Her husband knew this, but when she came home with some savings, they had decided to have another child.) And Thaton, the river port for Fang district, is a smuggling center, partly controlled by remnants of the Chinese Nationalist Army, the Kuomintang, who run the trade through corruption of local authorities, intimidation, trafficking and heroin revenues. I knew none of this when I first visited, and little about an obvious, burning question: why here? Why now? Why should a remote farming town have so many families like the one I met on that first trip? The answer, at least in part, is that Fang, and many communities like it, is no backwater as far as HIV is concerned. In the battle against the virus, places like Fang are on the front line.

It would probably be impossible to count all the wars, struggles, and challenges faced by the people of Southeast Asia in their long history. The latest is more potent than the cannons of the Portuguese, more insidious than the British regiments that marched through Burma and Malaysia, slower but more lasting than the American bombers that devastated Laos, Cambodia, and Vietnam. The next Indochinese war may be fought not on the streets or in the jungles, but in the blood of its people. The human immunodeficiency virus has exploded in Southeast Asia, from Burma to Vietnam, Yunnan to Bali; in farming districts like Fang, and in cities from Bombay to Saigon. It is already too late, as a former Prime Minister of Thailand remarked in 1995, for early prevention. It is already too late for millions of men and women in the cities, towns, and villages of the Thais, Burmese, Khmers. For the people of Southeast Asia the war in the blood has begun.

Where will it lead?

Recent advances in biology have led us to new depths of understanding of the molecular basis of disease. The HIV virus is known at a level of structural and functional detail unimaginable to Pasteur, much less the Sabin and Salk generation of researchers. In the last several years we have seen an extraordinary transformation in AIDS care: new assays to measure responses to anti-viral drugs, whole new classes of drugs to treat AIDS and its complications, combination therapies effective enough to generate, for the first time since the epidemic began, real hope for infected persons with access to them. Both basic and clinical research advances have been remarkable. In the same period, however, HIV spread has accelerated worldwide; the dense populations of Asia have proven terribly vulnerable. While we have come tremendously far in our understanding, the global HIV epidemic has leapt ahead of our best efforts. And, it bears saying, the overwhelming majority of infected persons are unable now, and are unlikely in the future, to receive the complex and expensive multi-drug regimens that are state-of-the-art care for the insured of the West. Only prevention will work for most of the world; prevention with what tools we already have and with those we desperately lack, most of all effective HIV vaccines. Implementing prevention will require changes in policies and national priorities for hard-hit countries. These changes, not new anti-viral drugs, are the best hope for saving lives in most of Asia. This is easily said, but not necessarily easily done.

Integrating new worlds of knowledge with the practical dimensions of health care, in rich and poor countries alike, has shown us not only what our new knowledge is capable of achieving, but also the inadequacy of our understanding of the ways diseases work in individuals and societies. We know much more, but we may not be able to do more. And many key limitations on the effectiveness of public health interventions have not been at molecular levels but at social and political ones. In the United States these limitations have led to painful paradoxes: we lead the world in understanding the biomolecular basis of disease, but we cannot bring ourselves to teach our children about condoms. We support and fund preventive interventions in developing countries that we cannot get past the conservatives and puritans in our own. Very different countries like Malaysia and the People's Republic of China find themselves in much the same predicament; political and social factors limit their ability to mount interventions. Communism and Islam may be wildly incompatible traditions, but they share ideological barriers to dealing with infections spread through sex. The Thais offer a striking and hopeful contrast. Burma and Cambodia reveal the harshest aspects of these interactions. Their health sectors are in chaos, their governments unwilling or unable to reform them. The absence of functioning public health programs has left their peoples unprotected from the full onslaught of HIV. These are tragic countries; both have talented and committed people eager to work on these problems who are violently inhibited from doing so.

What outcome can be expected in countries with large-scale epidemics of HIV? Population modeling studies, if we accept their premises, suggest that AIDS will not de-populate countries with high birth rates and expanding populations – just those kinds of societies where HIV is spreading fastest. But it will have devastating social effects nevertheless. This is a virus which preferentially attacks young adults, men and women of working age and women of childbearing age. In countries like Uganda, where HIV has been epidemic longest, the effects of this pattern of spread can already be seen. The middle generation, which traditionally raised the young and cared for the aged, has been depleted. With parents and breadwinners gone, children lag in education, health, and survival, whether they have the virus or not. The elderly suffer in poverty and isolation, attempting to raise another generation in late life. Education suffers. Development suffers. It could be argued that where HIV has affected the educated and mobile young, as in the Great Lakes Region of Africa, democratic trends are weakened. The young adults that Southeast Asia will lose are just the people these countries cannot afford to be without; a generation of young people needed to achieve prosperity and peace.

It need not be so.

We know from countries as diverse as Australia, the Netherlands, and now Thailand, that HIV prevention works, even in capitals of sexual activity and drug use like Amsterdam and Sydney. In 15 years of HIV circulation, the Dutch have had a national total of just over 5,000 infections – less than many small Asian cities have seen in just a few short years, less than many American cities (current estimates are that the US probably has 40,000 new HIV infections per year). In the Thai case, aggressive national promotion of condom use has led to real declines in new HIV infections. But condom promotion is politically sensitive in many countries, and even in Thailand, condoms are not available in some settings, notably prisons. Political leaders and the pressure groups they respond to have argued that such policies protect morals, values, national character. In fact they protect the virus.

Public health, wrote one of its founders, the 19th-century German hygienist Rudolph Virchow, is the union of politics and medicine.

Virchow's observation held true for 'social' diseases in the past, like syphilis, and social scourges linked to behavior, like laudanum addiction. HIV has slipped into an old groove. Understanding it demands an investigation into more than viral dynamics or immune responses. Studies of HIV and AIDS are likely to be incomplete not only if we leave out the medicine or the politics, but also if we neglect the status of women, the economics of the narcotics trade, the levels of social tolerance or political repression in society. AIDS has forced Western societies to confront homophobia, bigotry, and age-old fears of contagion long buried in the modern psyche. In Africa the reality of women's oppression, their poverty and illiteracy, have proven almost insurmountable barriers to AIDS control. Bad government and resultant social chaos, as in Mobuto's Zaire, in devastated Uganda, and in the murderous sister states of Rwanda and Burundi, have added exponentially to the problem. The very rapid spread of HIV in Southeast Asia has brought about a re-examination of traditional sexual cultures, of the social costs of rapid growth and change, and of the ways repressive political regimes have created national vulnerabilities to HIV. Nature abhors a vacuum, and viruses will spread wherever conditions suit their biology.

The virus forces us to look objectively at sex, and at the ways in which sexual activity often, even regularly, violates social norms and challenges shared mythologies. The Thais, for example, have a cherished cultural value of female virginity before marriage, and fidelity after it. How does this square with their equally long tradition of prostitution? Before the HIV epidemic this was an issue of interest to a handful of scholars, to a small group of relatively elite Thai women concerned with feminism, and, of course, to women trafficked into sex work. Once HIV entered this vulnerable population, however, it became clear that the majority of Thai men, married and unmarried, patronized sex workers, and the sexual behaviors of these men became an issue for all Thais. Governments, indeed societies as a whole, can be uncomfortable with these realities, and can refuse, as so many American leaders have refused, to see beyond their fixed assumptions of what constitutes 'normal' sexual behavior and to look at what people in their societies, indeed they themselves, actually do. This kind of rigidity can lead to disaster, especially with a disease like AIDS, where the incubation is long enough to deny that an HIV problem exists until the virus has thoroughly seeded a population.

Thus we heard the Indian Minister of Health in 1993 stating that 'traditional Indian family values' were the best protection for India against AIDS, not condoms, or STD care, or the protection of sex workers. But, of course, prostitution is a traditional Indian institution, with a religious wrapping,[4] high rates of patronage among young men, and a modern trafficking system involving neighboring countries, notably Nepal. The official insistence that Indian men 'just don't do such things' has lasted long enough for HIV to be out of control among sex workers, their clients, and predictably, their clients' wives, altogether as many as five million people by 1996.

If prevention works and is cost-effective, why has it been so problematic to implement? A short list of essential elements in the fight against AIDS might include condom promotion and distribution, improved detection and management of sexually transmitted diseases, access to clean syringes and needles for injecting drug users, rigorous screening of blood and blood products, widespread implementation of universal precautions in medical settings, broad public education campaigns and targeted interventions for those at highest risk. Getting these elements into place and functioning can be done, given availability of resources, but doing so may require several other factors: creativity; political will; access to education; freedom of information, expression and thought; the empowerment of women. It is in these less tangible realms that countries are likely to succeed or fail. The price of such failures will be high. In Fang, coffin makers are doing well these days: Highway 107 sports many. And a new class of children, *luk AID*, the AIDS children, have come into being. War orphans, if you will: survivors. They are relatively fortunate, given the prosperity of Thailand when set against the poverty of her neighbors. The future is likely to be unkind to the *luk AID* of Rangoon or Phnom Penh. It need not be so.

Notes

1. The project, 'Preparations for AIDS Vaccine Evaluations' or PAVE, was part of an international initiative funded by the US National Institutes of Health. The Thai PAVE was a collaboration between Chiang Mai University, Johns Hopkins University, the Thai Ministry of Public Health, and the Thai Army Medical Corps. Its purpose was to lay the foundation for possible HIV vaccine trials, a process involving the identification and characterization of people at risk of HIV (but uninfected) who might agree to participation in a vaccine trial. Other

PAVE sites included several US cities (Philadelphia, Baltimore, San Francisco, Seattle, and Denver), and sites in India, Haiti, Malawi, Uganda, Rwanda, Kenya, and Zimbabwe. My position, through Johns Hopkins, was Field Director of the Thai PAVE site.

2. The *wai* is the traditional gesture of greeting and respect in Thailand. The hands are placed palms together and raised to the forehead. It is done with a slight bow and wide smile.

3. Incidence refers to new infection or disease in a previously well person. In Fang we followed about 50 HIV-negative men with known 'risk behaviors' like regular use of prostitutes, a history of recent gonorrhea or syphilis, injecting drug use. None of these men became HIV infected in two years of follow up (1993–95); a result which surprised us all and which says volumes for the quality of counseling and HIV prevention the Fang staff were doing. But to identify those 50 negative men we had screened many more; over a third were HIV infected. We also tried to study sex workers in Fang; too few were HIV-negative to justify a study there.

4. In the traditional *devadasi* system young Indian women are 'married' to temple gods and then serve as temple prostitutes. Recent studies of this system have suggested that it enables women to be trafficked into prostitution by lowering social stigma through a religious affiliation. (Stephens, and Mawar, both at the X International Conference on AIDS, Yokohama, August 1994.)

2. Thailand: the descending Buddha

No condom, no service, no refund.

To the wide range of Buddha images found in Asia, the Thais have added only one unique figure. Sometimes called the 'Walking Buddha', the image is actually the Buddha descending back into the material world after instructing his first disciple, his late mother Queen Maya, in the seventh Buddhist heaven. The descending Buddha arose in Sukhothai, the first kingdom in the region that is distinctly theirs. The Thais had migrated out of Yunnan and into the flood plain of the Chao Phraya river only a few hundred years before. They came to a region long settled and controlled by the waning Khmer and Mon kingdoms. The late Khmer style had evolved into a kind of Hindu/Buddhist rococo, with elaborate decorative carvings encrusting virtually every inch of their corncob *prangs* (the towers that adorn Khmer monuments). Their Buddha was a solid, broad-chested man, with a knowing smile and a wrestler's thick face and neck. The Thais, once they overcame their Khmer overlords, created a radically simplified style. The change is as abrupt as that from the gilt and glitter of high renaissance Catholicism to the austerity of the early Protestants. The new Thai Buddha, having left the celestial realms of Khmer iconography, steps lightly back into the world of the flesh. Because they saw the enlightened one as having overcome all contradictions, all conflicts, he is an androgyne, with curvaceous hips, the suggestion of breasts under his monastic robe, a face that is both male and female, or neither, and of surpassing beauty. The Sukhothai form is all fluidity, in stone or bronze, all smooth curves with almost no decoration to mar the sinuous lines. The hands flow into flame-like points, the face is serenely present, the stomach, when it is shown, is completely human, with careful and oddly touching attention paid to the navel.

This image is the origin of Thai classical art. Once rich, the Thais quickly covered their images in gold and decorative filigree. But the Sukhothai root is there, in the best of their design and art. It is an image that helps define the Thais' unique sensibility and culture. There is the love of beauty, the acceptance of the physical, a shared celebration of the sensuous and the spiritual, the practicality of an enlightened being who leaves the heavens for the fields of the material.

The speed and vigor with which the Thais overthrew the Khmers and established a new kingdom, a new style of art and architecture, was remarkable. This ability to consolidate, to adapt, and to make amazingly rapid social changes is with the Thais still. It is perhaps one of the reasons that they alone among all the states of Asia avoided European colonial rule, deftly avoided devastation by the Japanese, and saw almost no fighting in the long Indochinese wars of the 1950s, 1960s and 1970s.

Humor, pleasure, beauty, love of wealth and ease, the delights of the table and the bedroom, these too are essential elements of the Thai way. 'Thai', in their polytonal, difficult tongue, means free. Thailand, Prathet Thai, is therefore the land of the free. This is not only an assertion of nationalism; it refers to a very deep strand in Thai culture: individual autonomy. For men especially, the right to live one's private life as one chooses, and to take one's pleasure as one will, is a birthright to the Thais. This is almost unique in Asia, where the prevalent mode in many societies is the submission of the individual to the collective. This freedom, again mostly for men, extends to sexual life. In the past, polygamy was openly accepted. While it is now socially frowned upon, having a second, 'minor' wife is common for wealthier Thais. As long as the liaison is discreet, it is tolerated. For private freedoms do not at all imply public acceptance. The public presentation of breaks in the moral code, such as homo-sexual liaisons, minor wives, selling daughters, is a social disaster for Thais. It is referred to as 'losing face.' To force a Thai to lose face is to make a fast and enduring enemy. But as long as a man's pleasures and indulgences remain in private realms, and these open secrets are not publicly discussed, no face will be lost.

This personal freedom, of shame as opposed to guilt (to use anthropologic terms) as the controlling social force, makes for a researcher's dream. If you set up interviews the right way, and establish an informant's trust in confidentiality and your discretion, people will tell you their sexual histories, or recount their past bouts of gonorrhea or syphilis, without hesitation. You can find out what has happened, what their HIV exposure is likely to be, in minutes. This holds true for men in the armed forces as well. In the Thai army system, being HIV-positive, gay, or even transvestite, are not grounds for exclusion or censure. On public levels however, things can function very differently. The Thais hold to their national myths with great fervor; they do not tolerate outsiders pointing out the flaws in their picture of Thailand, the wide discrepancies between national identity and gritty reality. Walk around Patpong or the other red-light districts of Bangkok and you may be shocked at how explicitly sex is sold. The gay bars with go-go boy shows don't pretend that sex isn't sold there, and the girlie joints are just as open. You can pay to watch people fuck on stage, see girls shoot hoops with ping-pong balls, thrill to a line-up of Thai farm boys jerking off. It's about as exploitative a scene as anyone could want, and all the staff are for hire. Yet Thailand was in a national upheaval when a British encyclopaedic dictionary (Longman's) included 'widespread' prostitution in its entry for Bangkok. Selling sex is one thing, making it public overseas is quite another.

Saying the unsaid, I have often had that awful sense, familiar to all lecturers, of losing an audience. Discussing data on northern Thai sexual behavior, for example, and pointing out that the numbers show northern Thais to be much heavier users of brothels than men in any other part of the country, I watched the audience glaze over with disbelief. If the numbers are believed, they are immediately blamed on the poor, the uneducated, or the hill-tribes (who are in fact too poor to use such services.) Bring up the same topic over beers, in a casual conversation, and all the northerners at the table will agree, with sly chuckles and innuendos, that they are the greatest party animals in the land. And of course, northern girls are the most beautiful; who could resist them? Why should one resist?

There were reputable medical authorities suggesting as late as 1985 that Asians might be genetically 'resistant' to HIV. The Thai epidemic later proved this thinking hopelessly wrong. But it was striking, looking at the AIDS map in the 1980s, that Asia seemed to be spared. Thailand was the country that first exploded the myth of Asian invulnerability to AIDS. This makes Thailand the logical country in which to begin an exploration of the Southeast Asian AIDS situation. The Thai Kingdom also has been by far the best studied, characterized, and understood HIV/AIDS crisis in the region, if not the world. And it is the country I know best, having lived and worked in Chiang Mai, northern Thailand, since 1992. Thai researchers, public health officials, activists, and people with AIDS have all been ready to address their difficulties, their work, and their hopes, with candor. And, although much of what is said here may sound critical, this exploration is also an attempt to repay countless debts to friends and colleagues, as well as to Thailand itself, a country I have come to love, even as HIV has led, inevitably, to studying its darker sides.

To understand HIV you have to deal with sex, licit and illicit, commercial and forced, oral, vaginal, and anal. This means going beyond 'cultural' standards and ideals of sexual behavior to study actual sex practices, however socially circumscribed. You have to look at the bleak realities of heroin addiction, the conjunctions of drug use and sex, and the role of trafficking. It becomes essential to find out what is not working within medical systems, to look for limitations, to understand inaction. This is not muckraking, but the science of public health research; investigating root causes of the mechanisms of disease-vulnerability and spread in communities. Some of these mechanisms are common to all societies, others not. Thailand is not necessarily paradigmatic for her neighbors; many primary factors that led to the Thai HIV explosion have turned out not to be applicable to Burma, or to Laos. But other factors and mechanisms are shared. And for better or worse, the openness of the Thais to publicity about the AIDS crisis has also meant that if AIDS has an Asian face, for most people that face is Thai.

Waves of spread[1]

By 1981, when the first cases of what we now know as AIDS appeared among gay men in New York and San Francisco, the virus had already spread widely in Africa, Western Europe, and the United States. Because of its long incubation period and non-specific early manifestations, there was little indication of how widely the virus had circulated or of how many people would eventually be affected. The virus itself was not identified until 1984, the diagnostic test made available only in 1985. Once the test was available, and it became possible to identify not just people with symptomatic AIDS, but healthy persons infected with HIV, the extent of the epidemic became clear. Perhaps half the gay men in New York were infected by the time we knew HIV was present. Some countries in central Africa were experiencing a new plague approaching Biblical proportions, with perhaps one in ten persons expected to die. These were the first 'hot zones' where the virus had been spreading in populations for an unknown number of years before an AIDS case had ever been described. Prevention of initial spread was an impossibility. Pandora's box had long been open.

Sporadic cases of AIDS also appeared far from these zones of early spread. All over the world in the early to mid-1980s, often in countries with very few other cases, men were coming home from Paris, Amsterdam, New York. These were men who had been part of the extraordinary international and interracial mix of urban gay life in the 1970s and 1980s. They were going home to small towns in the States, back to places like Thailand, often ill and often alone. The first known case of AIDS in Thailand occurred among just such a man, diagnosed in Bangkok in 1984. The patient was a Thai gay man who had had a long-term Western lover. He had come back to Thailand after his partner's death. His physician, Dr Praphan Phanupak, had trained in the US, and was one of the few Thai doctors to have seen AIDS cases before. Fortunately, Dr Praphan knew what he was looking at when his case first appeared. His patient did not live long. As far as is known, his would remain an isolated case, a spill-over of the gay epidemic in the West, a dead end for the virus.

The second case was identified in 1985. This was a 20-year-old Thai man who had *not* lived abroad. He was employed in a gay bar in Bangkok; a male sex worker (in local terminology an 'off boy': the customers have to pay to take him off premises) who had had multiple male and female, Thai and European sex partners during the 12 months before his infection was identified. This young man was probably one of the earliest cases of HIV acquired in the country. His is the first documented case of what researchers in the field think of as the first wave of the Thai epidemic. Several studies of male sex workers shortly thereafter made it clear that HIV was indeed spreading among these men and boys and, presumably, their clients and other partners. The other partners were mostly their wives and girlfriends, the majority of these men being heterosexual outside the bars and clubs.

The commercial scene for male–male sex in Thailand, in contrast to the extensive heterosexual one, has been limited to a handful of 'gay' spots in the country: Bangkok, the beach resorts of Pattaya, Phuket, and Hat Yai, and Chiang Mai City in the far north. While the men in the trade were, and remain, at very high risk of HIV infection, their numbers have never been large compared to those of women selling sex. Chiang Mai has 12–20 gay bars with a total population of perhaps 100–200 male sex workers at any given time. Add together all the brothels, bars, restaurants, Karaoke lounges and massage parlors where straight sex is sold and it soon becomes clear that female sex workers outnumber men by at least 25 to 1, if not more. The social and sexual network to which male sex workers belong is limited to perhaps a few thousand people. The spread of HIV among these young men was a personal disaster for them, a cause for concern for the health-care community, but not, at least then, a cause of concern for the larger society. In fact, there is little evidence that this network was involved in the explosion to come.

The Thai Government, through its Ministry of Public Health, responded to the arrival of HIV by setting up a surveillance system. Sentinel groups like sex workers, soldiers, and injecting drug users were screened for HIV every six months, starting in 14 towns and cities in 1989. Several earlier surveys had also been done by hospital or university groups. The information from these data would later be critical for understanding what was about to occur. Injecting drug users in the West were hit early and hard by HIV, principally because they shared injection equipment. Thailand was once a major heroin producer, and while this was no longer the case by the late 1980s, the country had perhaps 50,000 injecting addicts in 1988. Surveys among injecting drug users (IDU) between 1985 and 1987 showed either zero, or very low (less than 1%), rates of HIV. Then, in 1988, a dramatic change was noted in Bangkok. The sentinel survey at the start of the year found about 1% of IDU to have HIV. By August of that year, 32% were positive, by October, close to 40% had the virus. Perhaps 5% of IDU *per month* were 'seroconverting,' going from HIV-negative to positive, an unprecedented rate of increase. This was the second wave of the Thai epidemic, and it dwarfed the first. What had happened?

HIV, like any microbe, has conditions for survival and for spread. It is an obligate intracellular parasite, meaning that it can only 'live' and reproduce within a living cell. (A living human or chimpanzee cell, to be precise – which we must be, since the virus is.) It requires the exchange of certain body fluids – blood, serum or plasma, semen, cervical secretions, milk – to spread between people. It is, fortunately, not infectious by any other route. It does not survive in water; cannot, as influenza can, spread through the air. It is not known to spread through the exchange of urine, feces, saliva, tears or sweat. When its conditions are met, it will spread, with varying and still not fully understood efficiency. But it is a parasite; it needs its host, a living person, to behave in such a way that another person can be infected. We have to do its work for it. A group of addicts sharing needles without sterilization between injections provides an ideal opportunity. Enough blood will be left in a used syringe to spread HIV if the syringe is used again soon; the virus cannot live long in dried blood. Such groups of addicts are not hard to find in a Bangkok slum, but it is prisoners who are most likely to share scarce needles, and to share them with addicts from all over the world incarcerated in the same jails. This is probably what happened, since the subtype of virus (in this case subtype B) found among Bangkok addicts at this time was essentially identical to the virus infecting drug users in cities such as London, New York, and Rome. Once this virus entered the blood stream of one addict in these needle-sharing groups, the others were being infected with terrible speed. Because the addict groups were connected across the city, and, eventually, the country, chains of transmission carried the virus far and fast. In a matter of months, it reached one-third of all addicts in the country. But how many addicts were there? How serious a problem would this be? Estimates varied, measures varied, but a general consensus emerged that there were probably 50,000 IDU in Thailand at the time of the HIV take-off, 40,000 in Bangkok, and the rest in smaller cities and towns. In very rough terms, this would mean that about 15,000 people had acquired HIV in less than a year. A large and frightening number to be sure, but how much spread would there be from this group to others?

With most cases still found among gay Thais, male sex workers, and drug users, the Thai epidemic in early 1988 still looked somewhat like a Western one. After the first two waves of spread, AIDS was still largely a disease of young men living in cities, men who engaged in behaviors that the great majority of Thais did not engage in, and did not condone. This was not Central Africa or Haiti, where the great majority of cases were among heterosexuals, both urban and rural, and where more and more new HIV infections were occurring among women and their infants. Asia still looked safe from this perspective, and 'Asian Family Values' were routinely cited as having 'protected' Asia from the fate of the Africans. This rhetoric fitted well with the region's startling economic boom, and again, 'Confucian' or 'Asian' values of thrift, hard work, clean living, and dedication to parents, family, and community, were routinely invoked to explain the economic miracle of the 1980s. The economic failures of Africa or South America were failures of values, or so it seemed, and the extensive spread of HIV was yet another example of what was wrong with their social systems. The Asian way was superior, even if freedom and democracy were not a part of the 'Asian Way.' This argument was accepted with remarkable ease in the West, even when it was made by a dictator like Suharto of Indonesia, or an autocrat like Singapore's Lee Kwan Yew.

This complacency was not to last. Women working in the sex industry had been irregularly tested for HIV in Thailand since 1985. Some sporadic infections were found, but they never amounted to more than 1% of women screened in any sample. Until 1989, that is. A year after the sudden explosion among addicts, a similar rise was noted among women in Chiang Mai. Again, the rate did not go from 1% to 2% in six months, which would have meant a doubling, but from 1% to 44% in six months, a figure which seemed almost inconceivably high, especially as sexual transmission was thought to be so much less efficient than spread from needle sharing. Other cities quickly confirmed the Chiang Mai finding, though none was to reach as high a level of infection. National rates reached 15% of women in the sex industry by 1991. This was the third wave. The social and sexual network of which these women were a part was very different from that of gay bar workers or injecting addicts. This group involved the women themselves, their clients, and their clients' other sexual partners. It would later become clear that this network included the majority of sexually active adults in Thailand; it *was* Thailand.

To understand what was happening, or had already happened, we have to turn our attention away from Bangkok and go north, to the old Kingdom of Lanna, where HIV may have entered the general population first, and where it would hit the hardest.

The Kingdom of Lanna

Chiang Mai means 'the new city'. It was new in 1295, when the King of Chiang Rai ordered it to be built for his grandson. The city was laid out according to sacred geography, a perfect square in the valley of the twisting Ping river. The city walls had four gates, each opening to the four cardinal directions of the compass. In the sacred, but not the geometric center, a huge *chedi*, or stupa, was erected, filled with relics, Buddha images, and protective amulets. On a peak in the first rise of mountains above the town, a temple was built to further protect the new city. This is Doi Suthep, and its central *chedi* was plated with Ping river gold. The inhabitants were a mix of Lanna Thai, a people descended from the ethnic Thai minority of Yunnan; the indigenous Lawa; and the Mons, an ancient Buddhist people from southern Burma, who had been brought to the north of Thailand in an earlier effort to civilize the region. The inhabitants spoke a dialect of Thai which remains the common peoples' language, a dialect peppered with Sanskrit honorifics, Pali terms, and the equivalent of thees and thous, archaic terms in central Thai that are still used in the northern language.

Lanna Thais are seen by their countrymen as quite different. If you ask a central Thai about the north they will tell you that they are 'soft' people: polite, graceful, and soft-spoken. Northern women are supposed to be the most beautiful in the land. They are fair-skinned, small-featured, round-eyed, delicate. These differences are not just the stuff of popular opinion. Population-level genetic testing (using a technology developed for organ donation) now allows us to compare populations and trace relationships between ethnic groups. The northern Thais, it turns out, are related closely to the Shans of Burma, the Lao, and the Dai minority of Yunnan. The central Thais appear to be related to Melanesians, and are not even close cousins of the Lanna Thais. These differences have a very real geopolitical past as well. Lanna was only annexed to the Thai state early in this century, when the last hereditary leader, a 14-year-old girl called Princess Dararasemee, was married to the central Thai King. Until the 1920s, the journey from Bangkok to Chiang Mai took several weeks and could be done only on elephants. Tigers made the route dangerous. The Siamese tiger is now thought to be extinct, or nearly so, in the wild.

If you come into Chiang Mai today you will see vestiges of the old capital. The temple on the mountain is still there, surrounded by dense green forest. But it is a city of concrete skyscrapers, convenience stores, condominiums, shopping malls, traffic, noise and dust. The ramparts remain in some places, and all the city gates are still there, though motorcycles roar through them day and night. Americans can have distorted views of this part of the world. We imagine an exotic place, mysterious and more 'spiritual' than the material West. After a while, you realize the locals see the same distortions. They see the city they remember, a city of tree-lined avenues, girls with flowers in their hair, temple bells and elaborate festivals of flowers, candles and lights. Bangkokians love to come to the north and visit this 'traditional' culture. They have themselves photographed in native northern dress. Somehow they don't seem to notice that the natives are all in jeans and tank tops, that the traffic is approaching Bangkok levels of congestion, that the air is blue with lead from the cheap gasoline, and that DDT has killed off all the birds except pigeons and sparrows. Modern Chiang Mai is growing too fast to catch its breath.

One of the mysteries of HIV in Thailand is that the center of the epidemic among sex workers, and later their clients, was not Bangkok, a city infamous for its fast nightlife, but here, in the more rural and landlocked north. By 1991, within 2 years of the rapid escalation of infection in sex workers, HIV was about five times as common among young men in northern Thailand as in the rest of the country. The fourth wave. When you cut off the upper north, the region we know as the golden triangle, the rates doubled again. It is tempting to blame drug use. Opium, heroin, the Vietnam era, more mystery and sinister exotica cross the mind. But the great majority of Thai addicts are in Bangkok, not in the north. The drug of choice for northerners, for which they are well known by other Thais, is not heroin but the bitter-sweet rice spirit called *Mekong*. Unraveling this seeming paradox was one of our first tasks in understanding the spread of HIV in this old kingdom. This is the kind of challenge that epidemiology was designed for.

Today, the provinces with the highest HIV burden in the country are rural Payao, Lamphun, Chiang Rai, and Chiang Mai, all contiguous and all in the far north of the country. The provinces lag in development, and are still largely agricultural and comparatively poor. In 1991, 10.4% of young men drafted into the Thai Army from the upper north were HIV-infected, while among draftees in Bangkok, only 1 in 50 was HIV-positive. Indeed, the upper north, with less than a tenth of the national population, accounted for more than one-third of HIV infections and almost half of Thailand's AIDS deaths by 1994. Working with Thai Army conscripts, a large population of 21-year-old men, has helped to unravel this geographic finding. Northern Thai men, we found, usually begin their sexual lives in brothels. Older brothers, or other relatives and friends, take boys of 14 and over to the cheap local brothels which are everywhere in the north. Brothel-going is a men's group activity; it is considered 'perverse' or 'dirty' to go alone. Lanna men usually end up at brothels after a night's drinking, on pay-day, or during festivals and holidays. We found a direct relationship between frequency of brothel visits and risk of being HIV-positive among the army conscripts. Men who did not go to brothels (a small minority, perhaps 15%) were much less likely to be positive. The factors associated with HIV among these men, in addition to brothel-going, were not using condoms, alcohol use, having had other sexually transmitted diseases, and having had sex with more than one other man. The heavy representation of northern women in the brothels, cafes, and massage parlors throughout the country turned out to be another key factor. While making up less than one-tenth of the Thai population, northern women make up more than one-third of the country's sex workers (although this is changing rapidly, as we shall see). What historical and cultural factors lay behind these behaviors? Why were northern women so over-represented in the national sex trade? What traditions were operative in sexual networks, in behavior, in the practices of the people of Lanna and in the status and treatment of their women, that had led to what was clearly a marked vulnerability to HIV?

For the northern Thai man in earlier times, having multiple wives and other sex partners was one of the privileges of prosperity. Minor wives were socially acceptable, and wealthy men might have several. Slavery was a part of Lanna life for most of the kingdom's first six centuries, and slave 'wives' were common for those who could afford them. Any children a man had with his slave wives were his to sell. The modern trade in young women no doubt has some continuity with this tradition. The current emphasis on monogamous marriages has been seen by cultural historians as an adaptation to exposure to the West; earlier northern Thai traditions placed little emphasis on monogamy as a virtue for men.

The social tolerance of Thai culture has also played a role in the development of sexual habits and practices. While social codes of conduct may be adhered to in public, and loss of face a compelling social control, Lanna culture has always allowed for a considerable degree of autonomy in people's private lives. This relative sexual freedom, at least for men, appears to have survived till today. The use of commercial sex services, highly stigmatized in many Asian cultures, is an acknowledged outlet for northern Thai men, the great majority of whom have bought sex at some time in their lives. Like nearly all societies, however, this sexual freedom applies much less to women. Social codes of female behavior strongly censure pre-marital sex, extra-marital sex, and multiple partners.

How then have so many northern women ended up working in brothels? Poverty is a driving force, and parental debt, especially from gambling, drug use, and drinking, is another. But these social factors are common throughout rural Thailand, and do not explain the over-representation of northern women in the sex trade. The social scientist Marjorie Muecke has suggested that an underlying cause is the old northern tradition of daughters rather than sons supporting their parents. Northern girls, under pressure to support their families, and often lacking the education and skills necessary for better-paid jobs, end up as commercial sex workers to support their families. This, as Muecke points out, is something of an ethical paradox. As a dutiful daughter, a woman sending money home is fulfilling her proper role. The fact that she does this in a dangerous and degrading profession only heightens her sacrifice. Yet such a girl is clearly living outside the social norm of chastity until marriage. Here again, social tolerance plays an important role in accepting these women back into the community. The fact that so many women who leave the sex trade can go home and be accepted in their communities is striking. However, this has had a devastating impact on these communities, as well over 40% of returning sex workers bring HIV back home along with their wages.

Could it be argued that in this context prostitution supports the institution of marriage? If a society accepts that young men are going to have sex before marriage, and that women are not going to do this, someone has to supply sexual outlets. The high value placed on female virginity, and the equally high value placed on male sexual freedom, virtually ensure that a class of women will be used for sex. These would not be girls of one's own class, or one's daughters or sisters, but in older orders slaves and concubines, in modern ones sex workers. One of the most difficult truths for many Asian societies to accept is that prostitution is a core part of their sexual and social systems. If HIV had not come along, the Thais might never have had to face this. India, for example, still refuses to do so, despite having an immense local sex industry, and, by 1995, the largest number of persons with HIV of any country on earth (over 5 million by 1996). What HIV revealed in northern Thailand is that the prevailing sexual mores, considered so much more 'traditional' and 'conservative' than those of the modern West, were in fact almost ideal for the spread of HIV.

Because the professional class of women who supply sex is relatively small, and their number of partners huge, they rapidly become infected with HIV, as we saw in Chiang Mai. Lacking education, power, and, in many cases, freedom, these women can do little to protect themselves. Once infected, they can do little to protect their clients, either, especially if men do not want to use condoms. The result is a classic epidemiologic situation: a highly exposed and heavily infected core group interacts with a much larger population, the predictable wave after women in the sex industry. In Thailand 80,000–200,000 women, depending our your source, interacted with millions of Thai men. The fourth wave was among these heterosexual men, among farmers, soldiers, students, fathers, husbands, sons. Between 1989 and 1995 at least 600,000 such men became infected with HIV. Thailand had undergone the fastest spread of HIV ever documented.

The next wave was both slower and wider, and was also entirely predictable. Men brought HIV home to their girlfriends and wives. Newly married women, housewives, mothers, pregnant women, fetuses, and infants were exposed to HIV as the men in their lives had become exposed. The virus had moved out of the brothel and into the home. This tragedy may have been entirely predictable, but has still been difficult for many to accept, so strongly had HIV become associated with prostitution. But there is mounting evidence to show that the great majority of Thai women with HIV have had one sex partner in their lives – their husbands, and have only one risk for HIV – his behavior, which they may or may not be able to influence.

Are there other explanations?

Genetic recombination

Some time during the 1970s or 1980s, we are unlikely ever to know precisely when, a man or a woman or a child in the Central African Republic, a landlocked country to the west of Zaire/Congo, became infected with a human immunodeficiency virus. At that time and in that place at least two strains of HIV-1 were circulating: subtypes, or genotypes, A and E. Both are now known to have been circulating among heterosexuals in the country; both caused what looked like the same disease, AIDS. The HIV-1 subtype A virus was widely dispersed in Africa, and would later reappear when HIV exploded in India. The subtype E was much more unusual, a virus almost unique to the country. (Subtypes A and E were found almost exclusively in Africa in 1988. The virus that caused the American and European epidemics, subtype B, was also present in Africa, but the reverse was not the case.) What we think happened is this. Within the body of one person in the Central African Republic, both subtype A and E viruses were present. Through the complex viral process of reproduction, a mistake occurred. The viruses recombined to form a new variant. This virus, also called subtype E (but later shown to be very different from its parent) had the outer components of the E strain, but the core components of the A strain. With the techniques then available, it typed as an E when you looked at its outer coat (gp120) but as an A if you looked at core genetic structure (genotype). We don't know how this occurred, but we do know that this recombinant virus, seven years after its introduction into Southeast Asia, is by far the fastest spreading subtype of HIV in the region. It is recombinant subtype E that has caused the heterosexual take-off of HIV in Thailand and Cambodia, and which is now spreading in Vietnam, Malaysia, Burma, China, and presumably other countries about which we know very little (such as Indonesia, Laos, Bangladesh and Nepal).

There is currently a major debate among researchers as to whether this is a 'super-virus', which will cause heterosexual transmission in any population, or simply a lucky virus which entered a vulnerable population (women selling sex in Thailand and men buying it) and spread opportunistically, as any other subtype could have. In other words, does behavior explain the lightning spread of HIV among heterosexuals in Thailand, or is there a component of the interaction which is essentially viral in nature?

If this sounds like an academic issue, consider the question another way. Why did heterosexual spread not explode in New York the way it did in Thailand, going from gay men and addicts to affect, say, one in ten young straight men and women? Was this due to behavior, to the much less promiscuous heterosexual male as opposed to the homosexual one? Or were we lucky? Did the subtype of HIV introduced into the US simply not spread very well from male to female and from female to male? If viral factors are indeed important, and the subtype E virus is spreading so quickly in Southeast Asia because of some feature which makes heterosexual spread efficient, than the long-feared heterosexual epidemic in the West may simply not yet have started. Thailand alone has over 4 million tourist visits a year. In the red-light districts of Bangkok, Phuket, Chiang Mai, and Pattaya, you will see men from every part of the world. It is not hard to see how a virus spreading among heterosexuals in Thailand could take hold anywhere and everywhere. When we look at the case of Cambodia we will see that this is already, in fact, the case.

Responding: civil servants and civil society

Dr Chawalit Natpratan is a public health physician and *karatchakan* (civil servant). As Director of Communicable Disease Control for Thailand Region 10, the responsibility for government responses to HIV in the upper north has been his. That the people of his region were hard hit was clear to Dr Chawalit; that responses were urgently needed was also clear; that he and his staff would be able to implement control measures, and to have some effect on dealing with the rapid and incessant spread of the virus was not. But it would be telling only half the tale not to describe what happened next, for part of the story of the Thai epidemic is of an extraordinary mobilization against AIDS, and of some hard-won successes.

There are fortunate conjunctions in life and work, times when the political climate is right for innovation, when men and women of vision find support in public life. For the people of Lanna, one such conjunction was the result of a national disaster – the events of May 1992. Thailand had been led by a notoriously corrupt government in 1991, that of Prime Minister Chatchai Choonavan. He was ousted by a powerful clique of Thai military leaders shortly after. This was a complex but relatively painless transfer of power from civilian to military rule, a process which was not new to Thailand. But then the coup leader, General Suchinda Krapayoon, announced that he was appointing himself Prime Minister. Popular sentiment was strongly against the General. Protests spread quickly. In Bangkok, always the center of action in Thai political life, students and workers were joined, for perhaps the first time in Thai history, by shopkeepers and small businessmen, members of the new middle class. The protestors demanded that General Suchinda step down and allow civilian rule. The military responded with force, opening fire on unarmed demonstrators, killing a still uncertain number. Eventually, the constitutional monarch stepped in. General Suchinda crawled into an official audience on his knees to be shown videotape footage of troops under his command killing students. He soon stepped down. A caretaker administration was appointed to guide the country back to electoral democracy. This administration was led by a widely respected Thai statesman, Khun Anand Panyarachun.

Khun Anand fulfilled his mandate admirably; elections were held less than a year later, the military chastened, the country at peace again. He was also the first Thai Prime Minister to respond to the HIV epidemic. He met civil servants and physicians and listened to their advice. He created and chaired a National AIDS Committee, and invited a dynamic social activist and family planning expert, Khun Meechai Viravaidya, to run it. Together they scuttled plans for mandatory testing and contact-tracing, and instead focused on the rights of people with HIV, and on prevention and control. Thailand has a large and impressive civil service, staffed by career professionals, not political appointees. Thai governments and regimes have changed hands a dizzying number of times since the end of absolute monarchy in the 1930s, but the civil servants stay on in the ministries, the universities, the public hospitals, and keep the country functioning. These were people who, like Dr Chawalit, knew what needed to be done about HIV, given the political will and money. With Khun Anand in power, both were forthcoming.

When the first in-depth risk-factor studies of HIV infection among Thai men were published in 1991 and 1992, they were unanimous in finding that unprotected sex in brothels was the driving force behind the Thai epidemic. Unsafe commercial sex was a clear public health target. But what to do about it? Under Anand, the Ministry of Health responded not by trying to close brothels, or to arrest sex workers, but with a national program to promote safer sex. The '100% Condom Campaign', as it was called, targeted commercial sex venues throughout the country. Condom use would be strongly encouraged, if not mandatory. To make such a step practical, the Ministry distributed tens of millions of condoms to brothels, massage parlors, bars and nightclubs. Through the existing national network of public sexually transmitted disease (STD) clinics, sex workers were educated in condom use. In Region 10, under Dr Chawalit, every time a sex worker appeared at one of the clinics she (or he) was given 100 free condoms, along with training in how to use them. Signs began appearing in even the smallest and cheapest sex venues: 'No condom, no refund, no service.'

But outreach was also required. Dr Chawalit sent public health nurses out to brothels to meet the women working there, the brothel owners and managers, the pimps, educating them and enlisting them in the fight against AIDS. The nurses, also civil servants, were the foot soldiers on the front lines of HIV control. Mostly middle-class women, they did much of the difficult daily work of safer-sex promotion, STD treatment, counseling, and handing out condoms by the million. Night-shift teams were set up, which visited venues during working hours. One team in Chiang Mai focused on gay bars, making late-night visits to every gay bar that would have them, handing out condoms to the men and boys, showing gay safer-sex videos, answering questions. Because sex workers kept different hours from most other users of public health clinics, Dr Chawalit and his staff set up a night clinic for sex workers. This clinic provided not only preventive services, but also STD care, counseling, and a safe place to talk. The government STD clinics began to offer free and anonymous HIV testing and counseling as well. These were staffed by full time HIV/AIDS counselors, male and female, to offer gender-specific counseling. I worked with these STD and counseling clinic staff for four years and I can testify that the successes of HIV prevention in Thailand are due largely to their daily efforts, working with one person at a time, to make sex safer.

When there were gaps, problems, or areas of uncertainty, the government collaborated in research projects to clarify key issues. The research effort in Thailand was almost unprecedented in its scope and depth. The Ministry of Health collaborated with the US Center for Disease Control in Atlanta, the US National Institutes of Health, the World Health Organization, Unicef, the Thai and International Red Cross, the European Union, and universities including Johns Hopkins, Harvard, Berkeley, and the London School of Hygiene and Tropical Medicine. The Thai Army medical corps established an HIV research program with the premier US Army research institute, Walter Reed. When I was leaving the US to join this effort, a colleague at Johns Hopkins joked that if you spread your elbows too wide in Thailand you'd bump into another epidemiologist. These joint efforts strengthened the knowledge base for interventions, gave focus to public health measures, and, importantly, measured their effectiveness.

In November 1993 our group was working with the Thai army, measuring the rate of new infections in the conscripts. Until then, the rates of new infection had been depressingly steady, each six-month testing interval showed the same unfortunate finding: each year roughly 1 in 30 young soldiers was becoming newly infected. Sexual behavior had started to change; this we knew from interview data. Condom use was increasing, fewer men were going to brothels at all, and more men were reporting sex only with wives or girlfriends. But HIV rates seemed unaffected. As we analyzed the latest blood results that November, something had changed: only one man had become infected in the previous six months, as opposed to the usual 12–15. Six months later, we found the same low rate. I was literally jumping for joy in our lab when I saw that the second round of blood samples confirmed our earlier finding. Soon after, other groups were reporting what we'd seen; by 1994, a short 4–5 years into the epidemic, rates of new infection were falling nationwide. This was true for virtually all groups studied except sex workers, whose behavior may not be under their control, and newly married and newly pregnant women, that large section of the population marrying into a high-risk pool of young men, and starting families with them.

Possibly one million Thais had already been infected, but the rates that had been so high in 1989-92 were now sharply down. HIV had seeded the Thai population, and infections would (and do) continue to occur, but at levels which suggested endemic spread, and not 3 per hundred persons per year, which, if it had continued, could have threatened the economic and social well-being of the country. Thank God, or the Buddha, for latex, that milky sap of the rubber tree.

The successes of the practical Thai approach were remarkable. And certainly they owed something to the cultural setting, to the people of Thailand, as well as to leadership and good science. Promoting condoms was not an attempt to restrict the sexual freedom of Thai men. The army had tried this approach – punishing men for getting STDs, declaring brothel-going to be in contravention of the army code – and it was a complete failure: HIV rates were unchanged. Condom promotion in commercial venues required the tacit acceptance on the part of the government, and the people, that while prostitution was illegal, it was widely available. This was one of the most practical aspects of the campaign: by avoiding a moralistic or legalistic attack, it allowed ordinary people to continue their sexual activities, should they choose to do so, but with greater safety and with the government providing the condoms. There is also that other ineffable but very real tradition of adaptability that the Thai people have shown in response to so many challenges. They were willing to accept the need for condoms, and to change that most difficult of all culturally specific behaviors, sexual behavior, and on a population-wide level. No other country has had such success with condom promotion or voluntary sexual behavior change. The only other analogous success would be the rise in condom use and declines in HIV seen among gay male communities in the West; a much better educated and sophisticated group, on a whole, than rural Thais.

This is not to say that the AIDS epidemic was not growing rapidly in Thailand, for it was, and will continue for several years of mounting loss before it even 'peaks'. But we have to keep in mind the difference between new HIV infections, incidence, and new cases of AIDS. It takes, on average, 11 years from HIV infection until AIDS develops, according to American and European data. Estimates for Africa are about 9 years from HIV to AIDS (the difference being largely attributed to the interaction of HIV and tuberculosis in African settings). Survival after an AIDS diagnosis is generally about two years in the West, less elsewhere. AIDS epidemics, when hospitals are full and large numbers of persons are ill and dying, don't start for several years after HIV spread has begun. By the time cases of AIDS appear in any numbers, an HIV epidemic will be several years old, and new infections with the virus already on the decline. This is the situation in Thailand today. There are many more healthy people with HIV infection than people with 'full-blown' AIDS. The AIDS cases and deaths are greatest in the north, and rapidly increasing elsewhere, but the actual toll of the disease is still not clear.

This apparent split, between infections and cases, is one of HIV's great mechanisms of evasion. It also points to the unfortunate inter-action of this pathogen with human ways of thinking and coping. Leaders tend to respond to proximate problems. The press needs disasters, overflowing wards, before there is a story. The general public does not respond to high rates of positive serologic tests the way most of us do to a sick or dying relative, lover, or friend. It is a testament to the Thai public health community that they were able to mobilize resources and programs for *prevention*, rather than wait until care was the issue, care that even the West can ill afford, and that until recently offered very little hope even where it was available.

There were to be darker sides to the Thai success, as perhaps there are to any success, but Thailand still looks very bright compared to its neighbors. There could hardly be a more striking contrast to the Thais' impressive society-wide response to HIV than the tragedies of Burma and Cambodia, where the virus came soon after, and where it still rages with few signs of hope.

Note

1. The characterization of the Thai HIV epidemic into waves of spread has been adapted from the seminal paper by Weniger et al. (1991). For full reference, see bibliography to chapter 2, p. 225

3. Burma: going to Myanmar, being in Burma

For a long time the state of Myanmar's children was perhaps one of the country's best kept secrets. Decades of self-imposed isolation, fabricated statistics and the absence of social research and journalistic inquiry had created a false image of social developments. ... In fact, neither the outside world nor even the authorities inside Myanmar have an accurate or complete appreciation of the very serious conditions in the social sectors.

UNICEF, 1992

Burma and Thailand share a land border almost 2,100 kilometers long, from the mountains of Thailand's far north to Burma's deepest south on the narrow and steamy isthmus of Kra. The Burmese and the Thais share long, entangled histories, old grudges and rivalries, and memories of great victories, occupations and defeats. They also share Theravada Buddhism, the Pali canonical language, and calendars and traditions rooted in the cultivation of rice. Yet it would be difficult to find two countries with more radically different modern histories. Thailand escaped European domination; Burma did not – she was colonized by the British and ruled as part of the Indian Raj. In the Second World War, Thailand sided for a time with Imperial Japan, officially declaring war on the Allies in return for a comparatively moderate Japanese presence. Burma was one of the fiercest and most horrific theaters of the Pacific war, immortalized by the British who fought there. After the war, Thailand moved steadily toward modernity. Burma soon plunged into a civil war from which it has yet to emerge. Fifty years later, Thailand has become an international travel and business hub, its economy growing at 7–8% per year in absolute terms, its ports and airports among the busiest in the world. Burma remains a closed, secretive state. One is an Asian economic miracle, one of the little dragons of the Pacific Rim;

the other is classed by the United Nations as a 'least developed nation', arguably one of the poorest places in the world.

While the military is still a force in Thai political and economic life, there are other, more progressive forces at work as well, and their power continues to grow. Burma's military remains, after years of struggle and sacrifice on the part of generations of Burmese seeking reform, an absolute and brutal ruling elite, corrupt, inept, and heavily armed.

The contrasts are stark and conclusions not difficult to draw. But coming to any kind of political resolution in Burma has proved devilishly difficult. The Burmese military, the *Tatmadaw,* is dominated by one ethnic group, the Burmans. Burma, however, is one of the most ethnically diverse nations in the world, with more than a dozen major ethnic groups and over 100 different languages or dialects. The complex forty-year Burmese civil war is also an ethnic conflict. Hatred and suspicion of the Burmans only deepens as the conflict continues, as the roads to peace and reconciliation remain blocked. It was into this longstanding political and humanitarian crisis that HIV entered and found ample conditions for epidemic spread. As nearly every aspect of life in Burma revolves around its political crisis, a look at the recent political past is essential to understanding the unique dynamic of AIDS in this troubled land.

Dialogue or devastation

In the early post-war period, Burma was high on the list of newly independent ex-colonies thought to face bright futures. Educational levels were impressive. The country's universities and medical schools were the envy of Asia. The Burma Medical Association, the first and oldest in the region, was already almost 100 years old and sported a proud legacy of medical innovation and rigor. The British had built an extensive railway system and the country had several excellent ports. While much of this infrastructure was destroyed in the war, there were foundations to build upon. The situation in terms of natural resources was even more promising. Burma had some of the world's finest hardwoods and was famous for her indestructible golden teak. It was the world's largest reservoir of jade and a major producer of rubies, as well as other gems. The vast floodplain of the Irrawaddy, coupled with Burma's ferocious sun, produced an almost ideal climate for wet rice cultivation. But the greatest resource may have been the Burmese themselves, a cultivated and literate kaleidoscope of peoples who were the inheritors of nearly two millennia of civilization; a culture of witty and critical poets, learned sages, philosophers, artists, traders and farmers. Burma seemed destined for prosperity.

But the British left other legacies in Burma as they departed; there were unresolved questions of nationality and autonomy for some of the larger ethnic groups. These were non-Burman peoples like the Karens, Kachins, Shans, and Chins, who had been the bedrock of the British forces in their war against Japan. The British military had been a virtually autonomous force in Burma, quite distinct from the colonial civil administration, a tradition some historians have seen as pivotal in the gulf between civilian and military structures that would later develop. The one leader who had succeeded, at least initially, in dealing with these complex issues, was the young Aung San. His murder, on the eve of independence in 1947, marks the beginning of Burma's descent into darkness.

Burma did not turn her back on the world immediately. Throughout the 1950s, despite internal ethnic and political strife, the country was a leader in the Non-Aligned Movement, and produced the first (and only) UN Secretary-General to have come from Asia, U Thant. But in 1962 this period abruptly closed with the *coup d'état* of General Ne Win. Burma dropped from the world stage overnight. The military has ruled ever since. Ne Win, a secretive, some have postulated paranoid, dictator, set the country on a new path. His 'Burmese Way to Socialism' was about as effective an economic policy as the '*Ju Che*' of another regional dictator, Kim Il Sung of North Korea. Despite the boastful rhetoric of Ne Win, Burma's health-care system went the way of most other sectors in the society: it crumbled. Between the loss of talented people to emigration, incarceration, and execution, and the drying-up of funds for public health, what many argue had been the finest medical system in Asia froze in time and then slid backwards.

There were repeated (and often unreported) civilian and student uprisings against the Ne Win regime, all of which were met with brutal state repression. The last major uprising, in 1988, was different, however, because of its scope and scale. This was a national uprising, joined by virtually every sector of society. It included students, as had all before it, but also Buddhist monks and nuns, civil servants, doctors and nurses, and even the long-suppressed gay community. The movement, known to Burmese as the 8-8-88 uprising (8 August 1988 was the date the junta stepped in and started its slaughter), was led by Aung San's courageous and charismatic daughter, Aung San Suu Kyi. She preached and practised non-violent opposition to the military dictatorship. The aims of this non-violent movement were simple: the Burmese had had enough of Ne Win's hopeless and brutal mismanagement. Democracy was the key demand, the right to have a say in their own future.

One of the longest-repressed peoples in Asia had stood up. But the army was waiting. It will probably never be known how many people lost their lives in the 1988–89 crackdown; estimates range from 3,000 to 10,000. Aung San Suu Kyi was eventually placed under house arrest. Many of her colleagues and supporters were killed, jailed, or driven into exile. But there was a difference this time: the world, for the first time in decades, was aware of what was happening in Burma. Ne Win was reported to have 'voluntarily retired' and the newly reconstituted junta, calling itself the State Law and Order Restoration Council (SLORC), was immediately under intense international pressure. This pressure, and the SLORC's apparent (and mistaken) belief that they would win, resulted in general elections in 1990.

These elections were the first chance most Burmese had ever had to vote, and to give their verdict on military rule. Most of the opposition leaders were jailed during the elections, and could hardly campaign. Aung San Suu Kyi had no access to the media or the people. But one by one, all the time in terrible fear of reprisals, the people voted with their hearts. Suu Kyi's party, the National League for Democracy (NLD), won an overwhelming majority. Burmese still talk about these elections as a kind of shared miracle. Everyone had thought they would be alone in voting for civilian rule. So intense was the fear of the secret police, Ne Win's vast net of informers, that husbands did not tell their wives, nor children their parents, who they were voting for. But they had done themselves proud. A Burmese friend once asked me what I thought about God. I gave some vague answer about truth or love, and he answered with great intensity, 'God is the right to vote!' That was the feeling.

But the junta refused to honor the election results. After the bloodshed of August 1988, the people took not to the streets, but to the jungles. The ethnic armies, joined by students and democracy advocates, stepped up their insurgencies. The civil war began again in earnest. Burma's agony was to continue. It is still not anywhere near a conclusion. Aung San Suu Kyi, now a Nobel Peace Prize laureate (for her commitment to non-violent political change in Burma), was released from house arrest in summer 1995. There was hope that negotiations to resolve the crisis might finally begin. But again the dictators stalled. Suu Kyi began, quietly, to rebuild her non-violent movement and the NLD. In June 1996 she called the first party congress since her release. More than 300 delegates (including nearly all the 1990 election winners) were arrested on their way to Rangoon. At the time of writing, some have been released. Those closest to Suu Kyi, however, were swiftly sentenced to 7–14 years in Insein Prison, Burma's most notorious. Two have already died, including Leo Nichols, an Anglo-Burmese businessman and Suu Kyi's family friend. He was sentenced to three years in Insein for having an unregistered fax machine. Elderly and suffering from hypertension and heart disease, he died after allegedly being interrogated for 72 consecutive hours without sleep and without medical attention. Despite recent military truces with some ethnic armies, the Generals are still not ready to talk.

Freedom from fear

The first HIV screening programs in Burma were initiated in 1985, under Ne Win. No cases were detected until 1988, when HIV cases were first found among injecting drug users in Rangoon. Thailand had also seen an early spread to drug users, in the same year, but Burma would prove to have a very different pattern of HIV. The difference had to do not with the route of spread, for it was caused by addicts sharing injection equipment in both cases, but with radically different patterns of drug use. Another epidemic preceded the HIV epidemic in Burma, and this was one of heroin use.

Before 1988 there were pockets of heroin use in several of Burma's larger cities. The bulk of opiate use, however, was opium smoking, and this was a traditional rural practice among several of Burma's ethnic minority peoples. The mountainous regions of northern and eastern Burma have several ideal climates for opium growing. The opium poppy, *papaver somniferum,* grows best in just such stony, moderate-elevation mountain soils. For decades some of the ethnic groups resisting the Burmese military had grown opium as a cash crop to fund their struggles. This was analogous to the 'war-time' economy of the Afghan *Mujahideen*, who also supported their struggle by growing opium in their mountains (to which the West turned a blind eye, since the Afghan struggle was against the Soviets). Other ethnic groups were in more complex situations. Years of warfare against the central government had left peoples like the Shans without coherent leadership. A chronic state of warlordism prevailed in the Shan states. These warlords were supported largely by opium revenues. Warlords like Khun Sa became famous either as 'narco-terrorists' or 'nationalist leaders', depending on who was talking. There were purely criminal elements as well, groups for whom the war was an end in itself; the isolation and poverty of struggle served their need for secrecy in producing what had become by the 1980s the largest opium crop in the world. Poor and isolated Burma, off the geopolitical map, became the world's single largest supplier of heroin, producing as much as 40–60% of the global supply. This reality was not lost on the US, or the drug enforcement agencies of the West, but they were remarkably ineffective in dealing with Ne Win, the SLORC, or the ethnic groups to curb production. The limited evidence available suggests that before 1988 Burma was a major heroin exporter, not a consumer. This was soon to change.

The National AIDS Program of the Union of Myanmar did not attend the Eleventh International Conference on AIDS (held in Vancouver, Canada, in July 1996) but they had submitted papers, in abstract form, which were published in the meeting proceedings. One bears some scrutiny. It is abstract Tu.C.2547.

Rapid assessment study of drug abuse in Myanmar: A Ministry of Health & UNDCP co-sponsored project

Ba Thaung*, Khin Maung Gyee, Bo Kywe**. *Yangon Drug Dependence Research and Treatment Unit, **National AIDS Program, Yangon

Background: Myanmar society prohibits drug use, but acknowledges it to be a problem. In 1988, heroin use dramatically increased. IDU has since become a major public health problem associated with high HIV prevalence.

Objectives: To assess the nature and extent of drug abuse in Myanmar; To create a database to support a Drug Demand Reduction Program.

Methods: Used multiple sources and UNDCP guidelines; involved 36 high and low risk townships. Conducted case studies on 2277 IDUs in treatment units (DDTUs) and 937 users in 33 prisons. Also taped interviews, small group discussions, informal conversations and observations involving 186 key informers, 672 users, and 32 small groups.

Results: Drug abuse prevalence varied from 1.7% to 25% of township populations studied. Of 1333 addicts registered in 1994, 77% were heroin addicts, 22% opium addicts. 84% of DDTU patients and 65% of drug offenders reported using heroin, followed by opium (18% and 22% respectively). Users in DDTUs ranged from 12 to 77 years; 88–99% were male. Analyses considered ethnicity, marital status, education, occupation, drug preference, reasons for initiating drug use, duration of use, freq. of use, mode of use, forms/dosage and expenditure on drugs, familial trends, legal involvement, consequences of use, AIDS knowledge, and reasons for seeking treatment.

The abstract is the haiku of science writing. You have extremely limited space in which to summarize your concepts, methods and findings. There is a world of information in abstract Tu.C.2547, if we unpack it carefully. The great pity is that we don't have the paper, and this is because the researchers (who clearly undertook a massive investigative project) who did the work were not allowed to attend the Vancouver meeting. The same thing happened at the Asia–Pacific meeting the year before, and at the Yokohama International AIDS conference the year before that: no representation from Myanmar, all talks cancelled, their poster walls blank. I did meet one delegate from Myanmar in Vancouver, a hospital official who knew little about AIDS and cared less, but assured me that SLORC was really a very concerned and good government. (A typical party functionary being rewarded for his allegiance with a trip overseas.) Whoever did the work you've just read, however, was something else entirely – this is some of the most detailed information on drugs to come from the government. Listen to the haiku and you can hear the drumbeats of catastrophe.

Title first. UNDCP is the United Nations Drug Control Program, whose methods have been adapted here. This is the 'rapid assessment' component, an epidemiologic tool to get a handle on the amount of drug abuse in a city, state, or country. Myanmar, of course, is the SLORC name for Burma; to accept the name is to accept the legitimacy of the junta; if you call it Burma, the Burmese immediately know where you stand. So UNDCP is working with the SLORC. Fair enough; their mandate is drug control. But there is a standing UN resolution calling for the restoration of democracy in Burma and for the transfer of power to the elected government.

In the 'Background' section, we have the first acknowledgement on the part of the government that the 'dramatic increase' in heroin use occurred in 1988, the year they crushed the democracy movement and assumed state power. They also acknowledge that heroin use has become a major public health problem. The association referred to in the phrase 'with high HIV prevalence' is, however, an understatement. Another UN body, the World Health Organization, helped the National AIDS Program to measure HIV rates among Burma's addicts in 1994. The result showed the highest rates ever reported among addicts worldwide: 74% in Rangoon, 84% in Mandalay, and 91% in Myitkyina, capital of the remote Kachin State on the Chinese border. Note that Rangoon (Yangon in SLORCese) is on the southern coast of Burma, Myitkyina at the northernmost tip, and Mandalay roughly midway between the two. The virus is everywhere.

'Objectives. To assess the ... extent of drug abuse.' Given the astonishingly high rates of HIV among addicts, their number is essential to estimating how many Burmese already have HIV, but the second objective is more interesting: to create a database for a Drug Demand Reduction Program. This sounds, to those familiar with the jargon, suspiciously like the US programs, always promised and yet to be delivered, to work on the 'demand' side of the drug equation, the intense craving of users for their drugs, as opposed to the 'supply' side, the narcotics industry that is typically seen as the foreign enemy (Pablo Escobar, Manuel Noriega, Khun Sa, the Corsican Mob, and so on). But we hear no more about this program.

As to 'Methods', 36 high- and low-risk townships were studied. This indicates the scale; it was a large undertaking. We don't know how low and high risk were defined, but we do know something about townships in Burma. The junta has been relocating tremendous numbers of people and communities. These relocations, usually forced, have been done to move people off land for development projects, to get the poor out of the cities and into satellite towns where they are more easily controlled, to clear villages and settlements away from sites of historical interest for the tourist trade. For example, the premier tourist attraction of upper Burma, the magnificent ruined capital of Pagan, has been cleared of its surrounding communities. The residents of old Pagan have been resettled, out of sight of tourists, in a dry, inhospitable area about 20 km away. These new towns are something like the townships and Bantustans of the old South African regime. They are often places of stark poverty and despair. The depth of this despair will become clearer when we get to 'Results'.

Do 33 prisons sound like a lot? And 937 users in these prisons? And then we have 2,277 IDU (injecting drug users, so we are talking about needle-users here) in DDTU, which we have to assume means something like Drug Detoxification Treatment Units. It is not spelt out here, but we know something about the alarming conditions in some of these treatment units from Burmese who've escaped to Thailand. Firstly, there is no treatment. Detox is cold turkey, without methadone or other medications to treat the symptoms of withdrawal. Secondly, these are not voluntary units, but are on a prison model. Many are 19th-century jail facilities. The central one in Rangoon has undergone its first major improvement after photos of addicts shackled to beds reached the world's press – it now has running water. Conditions outside the capital may in some cases be even worse.

Now let us consider the 'Results'. 'Drug abuse prevalence varied from 1.7% to 25% of township populations studied.' This took considerable courage to admit. If, in any part of the country, 25% of a township population is using heroin, you have an unprecedented addiction problem. This is 1 in 4 people. This means every family, every household. If most of the addicts are men, as we find out a few sentences later, then this also means something like half the men in some townships are using heroin. And remember, the HIV rate in addicts in Myanmar is the highest in the world. Look at the age range in the treatment centers, 'from 12 to 77 years ...' Another act of courage. This is not a normal heroin and opium use population. Twelve-year-old heroin addicts are rare in any country; 77-year-old addicts are unheard of. This age range suggests populations and communities where heroin addiction is as common as drinking coffee or tea. And then we see that 88–99% of addicts were men. This is not unusual, but it does also show that 1–12% of addicts were women, and 12% is high in Asian countries, where heroin addiction and drug use in general among women is rare. (The National AIDS Program estimated that in 1995 perhaps 1–2% of all adult men in Burma were heroin users, and 0.5% of adult women. An earlier NAP estimate, deemed too politically sensitive by military censors, was that 4% of men and 2% of women were using heroin nationwide.)

The brand name for heroin sold on the streets of Burma in 1988 was 'freedom from fear'. This was also the slogan of the democracy movement, and the title of Aung San Suu Kyi's book of essays on democracy and freedom. What did the junta make available instead of real freedom from real fear? A deluge of cheap and widely available heroin flooded Burma after SLORC took control in 1988, and they have confirmed this with the publication we've just gone through. Is the SLORC directly involved in heroin availability? If not, they have managed to control every aspect of life in the country, every sector of the economy, save the most profitable one.

A student veteran of the 1988 movement now living in exile had this to say about heroin and the junta:

> If you put up a poster about democracy at Rangoon University you get 15 years in jail. If you hold a meeting to discuss human rights you get 15 years in jail. But you can sell heroin in the college dormitory and nobody will bother you.

Out of control

Heroin addiction does not necessarily lead to HIV infection: needle-sharing does. When the SLORC assumed state control and began their systematic repression of the 1988 movement, they closed the country as Ne Win had done in 1962. Foreign investors mostly stayed away (with the exceptions of China and some Thai military investors who bailed the SLORC out of its initial financial shortages). There was very little medical equipment available, and what there was largely went to the army. Furthermore, having injection equipment in Burma is illegal (as it is in parts of the US, the so-called 'paraphernalia laws'). The outcome of these events and shortages was the development of a uniquely Burmese heroin culture revolving around the tea stall. Every hamlet in the country has tea stalls, traditional places for people to gather, drink volumes of Burma's strong black tea, and discuss the events of the day (except political ones). Because needles were, and are, so scarce in some parts of the country, the tea stalls became local injection stations. Addicts go as often as they need through the day or week to get their heroin doses from professional 'injectors', working in the backs of the stalls, or some-where nearby. These injectors often have only one or a handful of needles; these are used until they are too dull to pierce the skin, and then sharpened with nail files for further use. Hence the extra-ordinarily high rates of HIV among these users. (Other diseases can also spread this way: a short list would include malaria, tetanus, syphilis, and hepatitis B, C, and D.)

In rural areas addicts also make their own crude injecting equip-ment, and these 'works' are frequently shared as well; homemade needles are sometimes made from ballpoint pens, or carved from bamboo splits.

The syringe and medical equipment shortage has not been limited to illicit use of these items. The medical system is also grossly undersupplied, especially in the civilian sector and outside the big cities. The underground Federation of Trade Unions of Burma has collected testimony from nurses working in the public hospitals in the 1990s, which paints a frightening picture of medical practices in the country. Surgical equipment is re-used until it is useless. Dis-posable gloves are rewashed until they're in shreds. Rubbing alcohol, a common disinfectant, was in such short supply in 1994 that nurses were diluting it ten to one with water; it would smell like disinfectant to patients, but it would not be of much use. The NAP admits that only 65% of blood is screened before transfusion – and even this low rate applies only to Rangoon. There are at least two states (out of 14) that have never done an HIV test, and where all transfusions are with unscreened blood products. For the insurgents, the situation is arguably worse. They transfuse in emergency conditions on battlefields where screening is an impossible luxury.

Since most addicts are men, it takes little imagination to see how quickly HIV could spread from the injecting community to women. Another UNDCP study found that over 80% of male addicts in Myitkyina were sexually active, and 98% had never used a condom. Indeed, of the 350,000–400,000 HIV infections estimated to have occurred by 1995, the NAP reported that 175,000 of these were among pregnant women attending antenatal clinics. Since the number of pregnant women in a population is much more easily estimated and ascertained than the number of heroin addicts, this huge number is probably fairly accurate. If the transmission rate from mother to infant is roughly the same in Burma as in her neighbours, and we have no reason to think it would be different, between 42,000 and 58,000 infants have been born with HIV in Burma since 1988.

Condoms were illegal until 1993. They are an unknown item to most Burmese, who have had only the IUD for contraception for decades. Condoms are legal now, but expensive. A packet of 10 from Japan costs 1,200 Kyat. The average monthly salary of a government worker is about 1,000 Kyat. You can also get black-market condoms made in Korea but sold in Russia (with instructions in Cyrillic). These are cheaper, at 750 Kyat for a dozen, but to buy them would still mean not eating for 2–3 weeks. In remoter areas condoms are something the educated have heard of, but rarely seen.

What about medical care for people with AIDS? The first report in the medical literature on clinical AIDS cases in Burma was published in 1993. These were patients seen at Yangon General Hospital between 1991 and 1992. Most were IDU and most were men. Nearly all presented not with the usual opportunistic infections seen in developed countries, but with tropical infectious diseases like salmonellosis and tuberculosis, a clinical pattern akin to underdeveloped regions of Africa. A recent article on clinical care for people with AIDS found that treatment was essentially non-existent, and patients succumbed quickly to infections. A Burmese doctor working in a government hospital in a provincial capital told me what she had to offer her patients when they were diagnosed with AIDS: tylenol when she had it and extra rations of rice.

In short, a health and human disaster, which will be extremely difficult to cope with in the midst of Burma's political nightmare. The murders, disappearances, and incarcerations of the SLORC era may be dwarfed by the toll in lives AIDS will extract from the people of Burma, though the responsibility for many of these lost lives may also be in the junta's hands. If this sounds biased, I must admit to being so. I believe that the democratically elected leadership could have done a better job in preventing this catastrophe and must be given the opportunity to try. It seems clear to me that the longer the SLORC is in power, the worse the situation is likely to be, in terms of health care, heroin use, and AIDS, for whoever comes to power after SLORC. And perhaps that's my final bias: I believe in the Burmese people I've come to know, and that they will win, eventually. Buddhism teaches that all wheels turn, all karma ripens, all regimes and social orders, good and bad, eventually go.

Being there

Myanmar and Burma. Two entities that can never be confused but which, unfortunately for the people who live there, co-exist in one time and place. Burma is a place in the heart where democracy lives, Aung San Suu Kyi assumes her elected seat as head of state, and reconciliation starts. Myanmar is an illusion of power akin to Mussolini's *Era Fascisti*, an illusion armed to the teeth, Buddhist Fascism, a seemingly unimaginable concept. Will Burma rise out of the realm of aspiration and be a nation again? This is the question at the heart of Myanmar; one cannot survive the *political* existence of the other. As for the two states of mind, both do exist now. The tensions between them divide the society like a mountain of razor wire, a barbed and bloody tangle.

The power of the Generals is everywhere and nowhere. Aung San and his daughter are also everywhere and nowhere. The battles are fought symbolically, in the heart and in the spirit, but the cost of capture is only too physically real. And they are wasting everyone's time. I have met officials who can't *do* anything about the AIDS situation because permission has not been granted. Talented civil servants scurry about their shabby offices like mice, waiting for the call, the fax, the message, that will let them do their jobs. (Civil servants cannot *send* faxes; they can only wait to receive them. Only the Generals send.) The Generals cannot be bothered, they cannot be cajoled; it is dangerous to reason with them. Their power is arbitrary, capricious, violent and absolute.

Rangoon is a city of deep poverty, more similar to Bangladesh than to Bangkok. The destitution of its people is all the more shocking because the people themselves, in their faded *lungyis*, patched shirts, plastic flip-flops, are so gracious, so deeply civilized, the inheritors of such amazing culture. You cannot help but yearn with them, for their aspirations; but also yearn to know them, to hear them speak frankly, to hear their laments, their losses and their ideas. The reality is that any such discussion could land someone in jail. Saying 'Aung San Suu Kyi', let alone that seditious word 'democracy', could cost one of these brave and decorous people their lives or their family's lives.

To kill time (already close to dead; only the Generals and their kin are going anywhere) while waiting for permission to visit hospitals and clinics, I was taken to the zoo. You could also call it the 'Yangon Animal Torture Center', or, to be more in line with SLORC, the 'Yangon National Animals' Re-Education Center No. 1'. It is all revealed in the eyes of one of four equally psychotic tigers pacing their few square feet of concrete. A Buddhist monk, a *sayadaw*, approached me as I watched a pack of deranged dholes (the small, red, Indian wild dog) pace in their dungeon.

'You are a visitor, Sir?'

'Yes. I am an American.'

'I am Buddhism, Sir. A son of Buddha.'

'Yes, I know. Are you from Shwedagon?'

'No, Sir. From a monastery here in Rangoon.' Rangoon, not Yangon, and said with a very faint smile. 'Excuse please, Sir. Are you contentment?'

'Well, Rangoon is a beautiful city, but your people are very poor.'

'Not beautiful! Not so, Sir! This is a war!' He said it again, forcefully, almost hysterically. 'This is war!'

'Yes, I think I understand. In my country many people know Aung San Suu Kyi, many people support her.'

Just then some people appeared to be walking toward us. Her name, and the people strolling within ear shot, sent the brave man off at a quick un-monklike trot. In a flash of maroon he was gone.

The truth of Burma is an open secret in Myanmar. Aung San, Suu Kyi's father and the founder of the modern state and of the army, is still on all the old banknotes. His face and her face. The central market is Aung San market, the park beside the old royal lake is Aung San lake. Everyone, *everyone*, knows who the rightful leader was and is. They have already rallied for her, voted for her, sat through six long years of imprisonment with her, and some have died for her.

After a day reviewing incomplete, but still disturbing, health statistics, I went to walk the streets of Yangon. At about ten at night I bought a *lungyi*, a man's sarong. The vendor took me to a side-alley tailor's shop to have it sewn closed. The alley was narrow, unlit, very crowded. About two doors down there was another small shophouse. A young Burman, handsome and wearing tennis shoes, so not poor, stepped out in front of this second store. At a signal I must have missed, a crowd gathered. They seemed to have come from nowhere, but in minutes there were 30–40 people gathered in the road, poor people, gaunt and ragged. There were several middle-aged men in rags, a wasted young woman with her infant, kids covered in scabs – hair tinged orange with kwashiorkor, protein deprivation. Three very old, bent Muslim men were called forward and hurried inside past the young Burman. The young mother was chosen, and several of the kids, roughly, with much shouting and argument from the crowd. Then it stopped. Others pleaded but were turned away. Those refused stood staring a long time before dispersing into the dark. What was going on? A work crew? A job offer?

I paid my ten Kyat for the stitching, (the official exchange is 6 Kyat to the dollar; on the black market it's 131 Kyat to the dollar, a difference worth noting) then passed the shop on my way back to the main street. Mystery solved: it was a restaurant, closing for the day and giving away leftover food. The young Burman had chosen well: the elderly, a nursing mother, and the skinniest children. But at least 25 people had gone to bed hungry. In my worst-case scenario for the SLORC showpiece city, I hadn't expected starvation. (This happened a few blocks from where the Thai Central chain is putting up a huge marble-facade hotel, close to the creamily restored Strand, where investors stay.)

In November 1995 there was a water problem in the city. No official warnings came out. I was having lunch with one of the infection control staff and was just about to drink a glass of water when he stopped me with the whispered word, 'Cholera'. Welcome to Myanmar.

Condoms are for sale from the betel-nut vendors. Walking alone at night, I am offered them on every corner. The Japanese ones are about a week's wages per packet. The driver the Ministry has loaned me makes 1000 Kyat a month, and if the car needs repairs, he has to pay for it. Most months, it is a losing proposition. Sex costs 5–20 Kyat a go. But men who partake can be charged under the British-era rape laws: ten years in jail and a ruined life. A virgin in the best hotels (for the Singaporeans, the Generals, the odd Chinese smuggler) costs a thousand US dollars.

Money is completely nonsensical in Myanmar. The notes are in 15-, 45-, and 90-Kyat denominations, since 9 is regarded as Ne Win's lucky number and the number 10 was deemed inauspicious by his personal court astrologers. Like the junta, money is also everywhere and nowhere. The Generals are not economists. Perhaps this non-system was the only one open to them, given their desire for both money and total state control. They are trying to keep a totalitarian political system alive, to maintain party control, but to have an economy based on foreign exchange earnings, tourism, international joint ventures, and the sale of natural resources. The result is a limpingly expanding economy, a new class of truly wealthy Burmese with state connections, no political freedom, and wildly uneven development. Health care continues to languish, HIV to spread.

The junta's biggest gamble, tourist dollars, led to a campaign called 'Visit Myanmar, 1996', and frenzied building of hotels, the forced removal of the poor from villages near sites of interest, and massive slave-labor undertakings to 'improve' historic sites. This had the distinct feel of Mao's Great Leap Forward, steel for steel's sake, with no real plan of what to do with it. So Rangoon has twenty hotels going up at once, unreported outbreaks of cholera in the streets, and a small dilapidated airport that will never bring in enough flights to fill half the rooms. It is central planning worthy of Stalin, with the same immense folly and social upheavals, which only add to the breakdown of the social system, the real local (subsistence) economy, the remains of health care, and family lives in SLORC's heroin-ridden new townships.

This disastrous use of investment capital passes in Myanmar for 'development'. However little it benefits the people of Burma, it can be impressive to the casual observer: big buildings going up, cool air-con lobbies and nice hot showers in the new hotels, Mercedes Benz's and BMWs appearing on the paved avenues. Visitors won't see the state of the schools, hospitals, and satellite towns. But then, neither will I, unless permission is granted, which is unlikely.

In upper Burma I met a doctor working in a hospital. He is a lovely guy: bright, committed, and brave. He is starved of medical news and information on HIV, and longs to share his work. We talked in the tacky VIP room above a local bar – his choice – a place supposed to be 'okay', meaning secure. He told me that in 1994 his superiors became alarmed at how many AIDS cases and deaths he was reporting. He was told to stop being so 'thorough'. His own practice has become almost entirely AIDS care. He is one of only two physicians in this town who treat people with HIV infection. Most of his patients have three things in common: they're young, they're addicts or ex-addicts, and they've worked in the jade and ruby mines in Shan or Kachin states. This doctor thinks the mines have been crucial in the spread of HIV. He explained that in the rainy season the mines have about 5,000 people. When the ground dries out, the numbers swell into the hundreds of thousands. People come from all over the country to work in the mines. It is dangerous and most don't do very well, but a handful do, and that's the draw. Heroin dealers are everywhere, as are cheap brothels; women migrate seasonally to try to earn some money as well. SLORC runs the best concessions; the poorest people sift through their waste water looking for shards. When the rains come again, the miners go home, taking HIV to every nook and cranny.

This doctor thinks the SLORC is not directly involved in the sex or heroin trades in the mines, but that there are corrupt people in the junta who are involved, and that their activities are tolerated because of kickbacks. The Generals simply do not care very much about ordinary people.

Health reform, like reform of virtually every other sector in this tragic country, will not move forward as long as the political process remains deadlocked. In October 1996, Aung San Suu Kyi attempted to hold another party Congress. The military surrounded her compound, and arrested over 1,300 people. The Generals still do not come to the negotiating table. Burma's agony continues; the triple epidemics of heroin use, HIV, and tuberculosis rage on.

In November 1996, a Dutch journalist visiting the Shan states discovers that people with HIV infection are being isolated in leper colonies. The leprosy patients are terrified of the people with AIDS, as are those with HIV infection of those with leprosy. This is reported to be a temporary measure. The journalist was also taken to see a new complex under construction, already surrounded with barbed wire. SLORC is preparing camps in rural Shan state for women coming back from Thailand with HIV. There is a name for places like this: concentration camps.

4. Cambodia: AIDS and the torn society

To make peace we must remove the land-mines in our own hearts which keep us from making peace: hatred, greed and delusion.

Venerable Maha Ghosananda

Phnom Penh, the Cambodian capital city, has seen more than its share of suffering in recent decades. It was bursting with refugees during the Vietnam war, then abruptly emptied of its citizens at the start of 'year zero' by Pol Pot in one of history's most fanatical and destructive social 'experiments'. It has been invaded and occupied by the army of Vietnam. Then, when the international community marched in, the battered city on the Mekong was, for a time, the center of one of the United Nations' most ambitious missions. Elections followed which produced something like peace after a bloody electoral process.[1] But the elections failed to end the Khmer Rouge (KR) insurgency and have left the country with a clumsy and ambiguous coalition government, two (incompatible) prime ministers, and a sporadically paid national army composed of several factions previously at war and still far from cohesive.[2] A violent and corrupt factionalism, scourge of past Khmer regimes, has hobbled the fledgling administration. A future of authoritarian dictatorship looks, tragically, to be a more likely outcome than the growth of a living democracy, the return of the rule of law. Cambodia's deeply cultured and creative people deserve better. But is hard to see or to imagine, given the current state of the country, how soon Phnom Penh will see the return of true civil society.

Phnom Penh *circa* 1996 is a *non sequitur*. Coming by land, as I did from Ho Chi Minh City, is jolting, a mismatch of countryside and capital that makes sense only if you keep the recent past of this pained and ravaged place in mind. Once you cross the border at

Moc Bai, at Cambodia's eastern end, you enter a landscape almost empty of people. It is pancake flat, the horizon broken only by the shaggy crests of sugar palms. The fields, or what used to be fields, are eerily empty, faintly marked squares of dust. The road from Ho Chi Minh to Phnom Penh, once one of the most dangerous on earth, has yet to be repaired. It is still not safe after nightfall, prone to banditry, Khmer Rouge attacks, or attacks by others (the police and the national army are frequently mentioned) often blamed on the KR. The hinterlands are heavily mined. What is most striking, especially after the bustling, intensively farmed Mekong Delta you leave behind, is the lack of human activity. There seems to be literally nothing happening: no farming, no trading, no mine sweeping, almost no traffic. The heat, dust, and silence don't give an air of peace; this is the silence of mass graves, of missing villages, of farms abandoned, of life stopped cold.

After a full day's drive through this landscape, arriving in Phnom Penh is like coming upon an Asian Las Vegas. The re-inhabited city is garish, gaudy, raucous, and thick with traffic. It is as though every car in the country, every building above two storeys, every fast food outlet, every bank were in this city. And there *is*, absurdly, an immense new casino on the riverbank, dwarfing the worn Khmer and French buildings around it. Equally bizarre is a massive floating luxury hotel moored at the same bank. Downtown Phnom Penh has a booming red-light district, spotted with brothels large and small, with Karaoke lounges and sleazy hotels, beer halls, and bars. It quickly becomes clear where the United Nations' billions were spent, and on what. Only pennies seem to have reached beyond the city limits. It's a despairing outcome to Cambodia's torment; crass luxury rising from the ashes. And more ashes for the poor. It is hard to argue that what Cambodia needed to rebuild after her trials was a casino, and not, say, a new university, a hospital, or some schools. Within an hour of arriving, I found myself longing for the country-side again, for that terrain of emptiness and sugar palms where the difficulties of life were at least not covered with neon and tinsel. Cambodia now is not 'news'; the UN has moved on to other crises; the fortune spent here is unlikely to come again.

Information is hard to come by in post-election Cambodia. Journalists are favorite targets of the new death squads. The man who appears to have taken control of the military and the police, and hence of the state, Second Prime Minister Hun Sen, does not tolerate criticism. His critics have a way of disappearing. Medical information is also scarce. Something like eight or nine Cambodian physicians survived Pol Pot's pogroms. There are almost no professors of medicine left to teach new ones. Health care in Cambodia is, by necessity, an affair of NGOs, relief agencies, foreign donors, and the UN. What scant information there is suggests grave problems, some only to be expected in the aftermath of longstanding social disruption, others perhaps unique to the agony of Cambodia.

As in the neighboring countries, HIV came late to Cambodia. Epidemic spread probably started some time between 1988 and 1990. As in Thailand and Burma, the virus found its requirements more than amply met. The origins of an HIV outbreak are ever obscure (and may not be terribly important, once local transmission chains are established and spread is under way) and this holds true for the land of Angkor. The virus may have entered the country across the Thai border in Cambodia's far west, where soldiers from both countries frequent a zone of cheap brothels outside the reach of both the law and health authorities. It may have come by ship along the southern coast where Burmese, Thai, Vietnamese and Khmer fishing crews work the dangerous, pirate-infested waters of the Gulf of Siam. This coast is dotted with small islands that serve as rest ports, fueling stations, and venues for R & R; the larger islands are also spotted with brothels. Many women from the 'boat people' era of Vietnam's diaspora work in these remote shacks. Without passports, legal status, or access to health care, they are about as vulnerable to HIV as a human being can be. Another possibility, which we will come back to, is an introduction from farther afield: the 20,000 young men who served as peacekeepers in the forces of the United Nations Transitional Authority in Cambodia (UNTAC).

The Cambodian National AIDS Prevention Committee is, given its limited resources, an impressive group. It is chaired by Ieng Sery Phan, a Khmer social activist, who has also long run the Cambodian Women's Development Association. She is a dynamic leader and has been able to garner enough donor support to begin to measure the spread of HIV and to focus on cleaning up the blood supply, at least in Phnom Penh. The committee estimated that in 1995 there were between 50,000 and 90,000 people in Cambodia with HIV infection, or roughly 2% of Cambodian adults. This is a serious problem, but it is the startling speed with which this population density has been reached that is more troubling. The prevalence of HIV among healthy young men donating blood in Phnom Penh went from 0.076% in 1991, or less than one in a thousand men, to 3.62% in 1994, about one in thirty. That is about as fast as a virus with HIV's infectiousness can spread, and suggests an epidemic out of control. These numbers, some of the only reliable data available on Cambodia, point to disaster.

Volunteer blood donors are an important 'marker' population. They are generally healthy young adults, as opposed to members of high-risk groups, and are usually persons selected to be at particularly low risk of having blood-borne infections like hepatitis B, malaria, HIV, or syphilis. Rates of any such illness in healthy people donating blood are more representative, and more generalizable, as regards what may be happening in the overall adult population of a city or country, than, say, rates among sex workers, or prison inmates. If we look at people from 'high-risk groups,' the numbers are much higher than the blood donors. More than half of all sex workers in Phnom Penh were infected by 1995, up to 1 in 10 police officers, perhaps one-third of soldiers along the Cambodian–Thai border, the wild west zone where cheap and unsafe brothels string the border like so many checkpoints. These very high rates are the stuff of headlines and they are disturbing, but the rate among blood donors means danger for many more people.

Cambodia today is not a society with the people or resources to deal with this kind of crisis, particularly as the effects of HIV spread will not be seen for several more years. The majority of recently infected blood donors are likely to feel quite well, and to be dealing with an array of pressing short-term problems: food; housing; security; rebuilding a life out of the ashes of the past; pushing, if they have the courage, for the return of civil society.

What seems clear from the information on soldiers, sex workers, and young men donating blood is that HIV in Cambodia is largely due to sexual transmission. While drug use is not uncommon, it is largely restricted to smoking the potent local marijuana, smuggled amphetamines, some opium smoking, and alcohol. The country is becoming a major marijuana exporter, and the drug is openly for sale in the old Russian Market, but injecting drug use seems to be rare.

Iatrogenic spread (that caused by unsafe medical practices) through blood transfusions and surgical procedures may be a bigger worry than drug use, although, again, the data are poor and scanty. We know that blood is screened for HIV in the capital, but the provinces and war zones are another matter entirely. These remoter areas are a zone of emergency surgery and transfusions, thanks to that most destructive of weapons, the land-mine. Getting information from these places can be life-threatening. One of the Khmer Rouge de-stabilization tactics is to kidnap and murder journalists, aid workers, and foreigners in general.

And then there is the war. Despite one of the largest UN efforts ever undertaken, and considerable international donor and NGO support, Cambodia is still fighting. The Vietnamese defeat of Pol Pot in 1978 generated a Khmer Rouge insurgency which has continued to threaten Cambodian governments ever since. Currently, more than two-thirds of government revenues continue to be spent on the war, draining the country of what limited funds are available for re-construction. It is a hugely complex and protracted struggle, and the original Khmer Rouge leadership still runs it. Imagine a quarter of Germany under Nazi control 18 years after the Second World War, and still under the men who orchestrated the final solution.

Cambodia is one of the most deeply wounded places on earth. You can see this on the face of anyone over 30. Much of the adult population suffers from post-traumatic stress syndrome (PTSS). An American friend, a psychologist working in Battambang, western Cambodia, from 1993 to 1995, told me that virtually everyone he knew exhibited at least some of the symptoms: recurrent nightmares, anxiety and panic attacks, flashbacks, irrational and extreme responses to memory 'triggers' of past horrors, substance abuse, depression, suicidal thinking, suicidal acts, rage. One of the most compelling symptoms of this national psychic wound was the well-described epidemic of blindness among older Cambodian women living in the US in the 1980s. There were several hundred cases of this perplexing phenomenon, near or total blindness among seemingly healthy women of Cambodian origin. Several hypotheses were investigated, but the great majority of cases turned out to be psychogenic blindness, blindness born in the mind. These were women who had seen too much.

Many thousands of Cambodians were Khmer Rouge cadres, and

thousands more have now grown up under the tutelage of men like Pol Pot and Ieng Sary, spending essentially their entire lives in the movement. Many have defected to the government side over time; the Khmer Rouge is thought to be down to less than 15,000 men in arms. But many, many more have served at one time or another, killing, raping, and torturing on command, often while still children themselves. National reconciliation in this tragedy means that these men and women will have to find a way to live again in the society they ravaged, that victims and torturers will have to pass each other on the street and not draw arms. Somehow the psychological scars of both sides will have to be healed.

It is a daunting prospect. Cambodia is awash with guns. Violence is used to settle even minor disputes. My psychologist friend in Battambang came closest to death not while the provincial city was under threat from the KR, but at a New Year's party. The next door neighbor thought the music too loud, and opened fire with a semi-automatic, killing the host. The thread that makes taking a human life difficult or impossible has been broken in Cambodia. The kind of scars that people here bear, and bury, have deep and powerful connections to the spread of AIDS, though these relationships are tangled, internal, difficult to investigate or illuminate. As Cambodia haltingly attempts to reconstitute itself, human rights abuses have continued, the use of force has not declined, the respect for individuals that marks civil culture continues to be undermined by the state. What is the nexus of these interwoven strands, a connection point between HIV and the internal nightmares of the Khmers? The sex trade is surely one.

Human rights and sex work

Trafficking of Khmer women and girls into the burgeoning sex trade has been increasing rapidly. HIV rates among these women are as disturbingly high as those in parts of Thailand, but HIV awareness, access to medical care, and condom use are all much less common. The use of force against these women includes not only forced prostitution, but beatings, rape, kidnapping, slavery, and murder. Contrary to the widely held belief in the power of economic progress to improve such conditions, these abuses are sharply on the rise in the new Cambodia. The Cambodian Human Rights Task Force, an

indigenous NGO that is struggling to get the new government involved in halting these abuses, has collected and documented a
heartbreaking array of cases. In March 1996, a fire in the red-light
district of Phnom Penh claimed the lives of two young Khmer
women. Investigations by the Task Force later revealed that the
women had been locked in their rooms and could not escape the
blaze. NGO workers interviewed survivors from the brothel fire who
alleged that the girls were under lock and key because they'd been
recently trafficked against their will, and had refused to have sex
with clients despite repeated beatings.

The Task Force has investigated other cases as well: in January
1996 in Battambang Province, a 13-year-old girl was beaten to death
by a brothel manager who had bought her for prostitution. She also
had refused to become a sex worker, despite repeated and worsening
beatings, the last one being fatal. This girl's story came to light only
because other girls enslaved by the same owner were so proud of her
refusal to submit to rape. One managed to escape, and carried this
tale of martyrdom to a teacher, who contacted the Task Force. The
owner paid his way out of a trial. Another young woman forced into
sex work died in a brothel fire in February 1996; she had been
shackled to a bed in the brothel to prevent escape. These incidents
are seen by NGO workers as part of a new trend in the sex trade:
kidnapping and forced sex work by organized rings trying to cash in
on the growing sex industry. The Khmer Rouge enslaved and killed
for ideological, if insane, reasons. Sex slavery in the new regime is
strictly a for-profit enterprise, but the methods are no less brutal,
and the outcome no less horrific. It is perhaps a continuum, and it's
not hard to imagine that some of the same people are involved. Was
the brothel owner who beat a brave 13-year-old to death a Khmer
Rouge torturer, or a brutalized victim himself? Almost everyone in
this society was one or the other. Neutrality was not an option.

Phnom Penh is becoming a busy place for Asia's businessmen.
This is another country, like Burma, where a significant chunk of
investment is from the newly rich Pacific rim states, and not the
West. Japan, Thailand, Singapore, Malaysia, Taiwan, China, and
Indonesia are all major players in the development business here. It
is an open secret that many of these businessmen want sex when
they travel. The rhetoric of 'Asian Values,' or Confucian principles,
falls flat if you take an evening stroll in Phnom Penh. The large and

sleazy brothel district has signs not only in English and French, but in Chinese, Korean, Japanese and Thai, offering 'full body massage', 'Karaoke with lovely hostess', a 'Good Time for You'.

The sex trade is not limited to the capital. Aid workers with the French medical charity Médecins Sans Frontières (MSF) working with women in the trade in the river port of Siem Riep, the gateway to Angkor, estimate that about 400 women are selling sex on any given day. (The overall population of the town is about 12,000.) Most of the business is local, according to MSF. The town is heavily militarized, and there are large de-mining teams, guards for the temple complexes, and many police. These men are poor and infrequently paid, but, thanks to the tourist and smuggling trades, there is some money in the local economy – enough to support a relatively large number of sex venues. Unlike Phnom Penh, where the trade is very much out in the open, Siem Riep is relatively discreet. If you're used to the way sex is sold in this region, it isn't hard to find, but the brothels don't line the main street. There are no real taxis in town, but local men sell rides on the back of their motorcycles. If you're a single man walking in town at night, these obliging fellows will immediately offer to take you to a girl. I never left my little guesthouse without attracting a steady stream of these motorized pimps.

The conditions in these upcountry brothels are abysmal. I spent an afternoon with Dr Else de Bruge, a Dutch MSF volunteer working with women and girls from Siem Riep's brothels. Her first challenge was education. The majority of her patients had almost no knowledge of sexually transmitted diseases, of their own body parts. Condom use had become a huge issue for Dr de Bruge, and was much more complex than she had imagined. She had been at the job only a few months, and had begun thinking the issues were ones of availability, cost, and cultural appropriateness. She had found out quickly that condom use was very low or absent. But it soon became clear that many of the women, particularly the Khmer girls, were too traumatized to begin to deal with negotiating condom use with clients. They couldn't even bring themselves to discuss these issues with each other, with Else, much less with men. Brothel sex happens in silence, in the dark, and most of the men are drunk. Most of the young women had no choice but to accept clients who refused to use condoms, even men with STDs. Else began to rethink her approach, and spoke in terms of basic development, helping women to understand their bodies, to speak about sexuality, gradually to take some control of the lives they were now living. Dealing with protection, with 'safer sex practices' as we blandly call them, would follow later. While condoms are the cornerstone of prevention of sexual transmission, they have to be introduced into a context in which women who have never had to deal with sexual issues can begin to do this. It means touching condoms, looking at them, consciously thinking about being with men, and about their bodies. This is a painful, slow process, especially for women who are, to use a medical term, displacing themselves, going into psychological retreat from reality rather than face the drunk strangers already inside their bodies. We tend to be rather blithe about introducing condoms, and medical people are particularly bad about this, forgetting how difficult it is for most people to be rational and neutral about the body. Condoms go on an erect penis. Obvious enough. But for a village girl or a returning refugee, sold to a pimp and trafficked to a town far from home and family, even thinking about an erect penis is a nightmare. And you are asking her to learn how to put one on a man who is, in a very real sense, a part of serial rape. Many women do learn to do this, but more than half will become HIV-infected before they begin to protect themselves. Condoms are available in the markets in Phnom Penh, but are too expensive for many local people – prohibitively so for most in the countryside.

The International Red Cross is also active in Siem Riep. They have had to assist more than 38,000 returning refugees to the heavily mined province. (The country has had to contend with the return of nearly 400,000 refugees overall, many of whom have been unable to return to their homes due to fighting, land-mines, or both.) In Siem Riep province, many of the returnees have become internally displaced persons, with fading hope of returning to their homes and past occupations. It takes little imagination to guess how vulnerable the women and girls of these families might be to brothel traffickers. A Red Cross officer in Siem Riep told me that HIV prevention is low on the list of priorities for the people of the province. He said this with great sadness; as a medical man, he knew only too well what was in store. He listed for me what he felt the priorities were in descending order of importance: finding enough food, securing housing, avoiding land-mines, finding a job in the still marginal economy, and the end of the war. HIV prevention (buying condoms, for example) can indeed sound like a luxury, given this plethora of basic unmet needs. It is just this inability to respond to the seemingly distant and abstract threat of HIV when faced with more concrete threats to life that has led to the most severe HIV epidemics in central Africa, where, in some countries, up to one-third of young adults may die. This may be where Cambodia is headed.

Official responses to the rise in the sex trade have so far been disturbing. In late 1995, three women employed in the sex industry were raped by uniformed police officers while taking an afternoon walk around Wat Phnom, an old temple at the northern end of the city. They were dragged into bushes near the temple and raped in daylight. The policemen's defense? 'Prostitutes cannot be raped because they are prostitutes.' The three women, with NGO support, pushed the new legal system for action. The officers were not tried, but were eventually fined token amounts. One of the people involved in helping the women raise funds for the trial told me that the most difficult problem was convincing the judges that a crime had been committed. The evidence for rape was overwhelming, but the judges agreed with the police that prostitutes 'couldn't be raped'. Judges, too, were targets of the Khmer Rouge, and most of the country's skilled jurists are long dead. Pressured to respond to the rising tide of rights abuses, deaths of prostitutes, and pressure from local and international organizations – particularly those that deal with child prostitution, such as End Child Prostitution in Asian Tourism (ECPAT) – the National Assembly began debating the issue in its 1996 legislative session. Rejecting calls for regulation of the sex industry, which had come from women's and health advocates, the legislators passed instead an order to 'eradicate' prostitution. (Eradication has unfortunate echoes in Cambodia.) Predictably, the order has had no visible effect on the sex trade, but it has made access to sex workers by their advocates more difficult and made the women even less likely to seek medical care.

A double lethality

Cambodia has another daunting challenge to face in HIV control: the small, cheap weapon that America, Italy, and China continue to produce to such profit, the land-mine. The Land-Mines Advisory Group, a Phnom Penh-based organization struggling to deal with the problem, estimates that between 6 and 10 million land-mines remain active in Cambodia, making it, with Angola and Afghanistan, one of the most heavily mined places on earth. Mine-clearing operations have been underway since 1991, and, given the difficulty of mine detection and de-activation, progress has been considerable. The Advisory Group reports that about 40,000 mines have been cleared since the operations began. At the current rate of 10,000 mines per year, it would take until late in the 21st century before Cambodia was safe for farming again, if no new mines were laid. But the laying of new mines continues apace. Both the Khmer Rouge insurgents and the National Army continue to use them along their front lines.

Each time a land-mine maims, emergency surgery is likely to be needed to save a limb or a life. Blood transfusions are also likely to be needed, again under emergency conditions. The current rate of land-mine maimings and killings is approximately 400 per month. Many of these injuries and deaths happen to children, who are among the most likely to wander off roads and beaten paths, to play in fields and forests. Land-mines in a country with high rates of HIV and limited ability to screen blood or sterilize surgical equipment may have a dual lethality: be killed in the blast or risk acquiring HIV. This may sound like an unusual scenario, but the people of Angola, Mozambique, and Afghanistan know about land-mines, poor or absent medical care, blood transfusions in tents, and lost limbs.

Men of the UN

Cambodia offers some painful truths, if we would listen. We can learn of the legacy of American bombing, of Nixon and Kissinger's secret war, the depth that a human being can be brought to if pushed early and hard enough, the speed with which a nation can be destroyed and the agonizingly slow process of rebuilding one, and what can happen when HIV enters a ravaged society. For the international community, there is another dark teaching with wide implications. There is considerable evidence that the HIV epidemic in Cambodia was heavily influenced by the presence of UNTAC. The UNTAC mission was the first of its kind, and to date the only time the UN has actually served as the governing body for a sovereign state. It brought more than 20,000 people from numerous countries, including soldiers from the US, Western Europe, Bulgaria, Uruguay,

India, Pakistan, Bangladesh, Thailand, Indonesia, Korea, and several African states. The great majority were young men, often of limited education. They walked into a country long closed to the outside world, starved for cash, and full of people eager to take their dollars. Prostitution was a likely outcome of this mix. It should have been just as likely that these troops were prepared to deal with HIV and other sexually transmitted diseases, but it didn't happen that way.

Local authorities are quick to blame UNTAC for the spread of HIV in Cambodia, insisting that prostitution was rare before the soldiers came, and HIV unheard of. This is taken as gospel in Phnom Penh's expatriate community, where tales of Bulgarian gang rapes and Uruguayan orgies with Khmer and Vietnamese girls are standard party fair. This is no doubt an over-simplification. But there is some evidence that the large number of international peace-keeping forces dramatically increased the demand for sex services. The infusion of cash from these forces into local economies after years of poverty and isolation was undoubtedly too great an attraction for many women (and brothel owners, managers, and traffickers) to resist. NGOs who were active with women in the sex trade before and during the UNTAC period report that sex workers, on average, doubled their nightly number of customers, from 5 to 10, during the UN mission.[3] Trafficking increased, as did migration of unforced professional sex workers from Vietnam.

The rates of HIV among blood donors in Phnom Penh also show that the 1991–95 period was marked by explosive spread of HIV in the general population. This was the UNTAC era. Whatever else we can say about the relationships between the HIV outbreak and the presence of the UN forces, they were happening at the same time and in the same place, and to the same people; ordinary Khmers caught again in cross-fire.

Soldiers from some of these countries undoubtedly came to Cambodia with HIV infection. Some may have been given HIV/AIDS education and condoms; other countries prohibit such education for soldiers, reasoning (there is no evidence for this) that such education might promote sexual activity. Muslim nations, like Pakistan, are notorious for these omissions. Other sexually conservative countries, like India, also resist such prevention activities. In either case, we do know that many of these soldiers left Cambodia with HIV infection. Studies of returning UNTAC soldiers in Uruguay and the USA have shown that most were infected with subtype E of HIV, which has previously been found only in Southeast Asia and Central Africa. They are likely to have become infected either in Cambodia or during visits to neighboring countries. Fully 15% of the Indian soldiers who served in UNTAC came home with HIV infection. This is an issue of more than academic interest. There is some evidence that subtype E may be more infectious through sex, and from female to male, than other subtypes. If subtype E has caused explosive heterosexual epidemics because it is more infectious through this route, then the global dispersion of subtype E from Cambodia is a potential public health disaster. It is a possibility that heterosexual epidemics in the West, long promised but in truth largely unseen, may now begin. It would be a tragedy indeed if peacekeeping missions, which the world supports for compassionate reasons, led to such suffering.

If there is any responsibility to be ascribed for this situation, it must lie with those governments which resist HIV-prevention programs for troops sent overseas. It is vital that future international efforts at peace-keeping, especially those of the UN, adopt comprehensive and frank HIV-prevention programs before such missions are undertaken. But the political feasibility of such programs is dubious, however important the consequences of not doing so. Failure to do what is needed on the part of the UN and its member states could make UN forces unnecessarily vulnerable to HIV infection as well as potential agents of HIV spread worldwide. Certainly, the outcome for the Khmer people has been a disaster. Khmer culture generally does not accept women who have been sex workers back into society. The large number of women who entered the trade during UNTAC now have few options but to continue. With Asian business activities increasing in the Cambodia, the next wave of clients has arrived to replace the soldiers. Prostitution is likely to be further entrenched.

One step at a time

Are there reasons for optimism in Cambodia? For hope? You find yourself asking this question almost daily in Cambodia. The kindness and sincerity of the Khmer people, despite the litany of challenges and abuses they have known, demands that you address it. While there is hunger in the country today, for food and for education, the Khmers I met hungered most for peace and for contacts with the outside world. Everyone I contacted for information and insight into the HIV situation responded quickly and positively, though many had cause to be afraid of doing so. This is a country where truth now matters intensely to people and they are eager to tell their stories. Conversations are long, food and drink and consideration are shared in abundance, criticism of the government is not held back. That generosity and courage could survive among so many people after what they'd known is more than inspiring. You come quickly to love the Khmer people for their tenacious belief in the goodness of other human beings. The young generation of Khmers who were children during, or were born after, the Pol Pot period are an impressive group. Walking the city, sitting in a tea shop, visiting a hospital or a school, you invariably end up in a conversation with these young Khmers. They want to practice English, but they are even more eager to talk about the future of Cambodia, their own futures and dreams. They are eager to learn, to travel, to help their country. While their concepts of democracy may be somewhat naive, democracy is the word that comes up again and again. Like the Chinese students of the 1989 democracy movement, what they want is a say in their own future, and what they are most against is the corruption of the elite. The nationalist rhetoric of the new regime is not fooling these young people. They know the real issue for most in power is personal profit. They want change. The country desperately needs reform, and it is these young people, not the UN, who will have to help bring it about. One only prays they can. They have at least one powerful example to follow.

The Supreme Patriarch of Cambodia, the Venerable Maha Ghosananda, is head of the kingdom's Buddhist clergy. He is one of the national figures at the center of Cambodia's revival of civil culture. Maha Ghosananda is a peace and democracy advocate, a social activist as well as a practicing monk and teacher of Buddhism. He is trying to bring about lasting national reconciliation through a revival of the spirit. His method is the Dhamma Yattra, the walk for peace. He has led six of these yearly mass pilgrimages thus far, going to every corner of the kingdom, bringing a message of *Mettha*, loving-kindness, to ravaged rural communities. The most recent Dhamma Yattra also carried an environmental message. Cambodia is being rapidly deforested. The marchers planted tree seedlings wherever they went.

Maha, as he prefers to be called by Western friends, is a man of

70, small and fit, his face a play of intelligence, compassion, and enthusiasm. I was granted an interview with him in Phnom Penh. I asked him first about reconciliation.

'I have offered the leaders of the Khmer Rouge, Pol Pot and his senior men, to ordain them as Buddhist monks. From our perspective, they have earned a large negative karma by causing so much suffering. Also, they are suffering themselves. They will have to begin to deal with this karma, either in this life or the next ones, so it is better for them if they start now. The sooner the better.'

'Did any accept the offer?'

'No. But they may someday. A good number of their soldiers are becoming monks. Many young men in Cambodia today are becoming monks, but I have to tell you that for most they choose ordination as a way of staying out of the army. They are not so serious about meditation. But it is still better than fighting. The *Sangha* is getting very big!'

'There is still so much violence and injustice in your country. And now AIDS has spread very quickly. I fear that the medical system will not be able to cope. How can your country be healed?'

'Suffering is a part of life. We are all suffering. But it is all right, it is improving, people are coming back to the temples, to the mosques, and beginning to practice mindfulness again, which is the only way to see through suffering. The government too, they will have to come around. And they will. Although suffering will continue. It always has.'

'When you led a peace march into the Khmer-Rouge-held territory, you and your followers were shelled. Are you worried about the next Dhamma Yattra?'

'We take one step at a time. One breath at a time. Keeping mindful of our actions, our minds. With each mindful step, we move closer to peace. This is the process and nothing can stop it.'

'I would like to come on your next march, but unfortunately I have to be back in Thailand.'

'Just take a few mindful steps with us, each day. It doesn't matter where you are. Khmer people are joining us in mindfulness in Thailand, in the States. You can do it in Chiang Mai. It doesn't matter.'

'Maha, tell me about Cambodian Buddhism. I've read that this is a Theravada country, but I see elements of Mahayana also. And much of Angkor was Hindu, wasn't it?'

'Yes, some of the people were Hindus. The names are not important, just the practice. In Cambodian Buddhism we have all three schools; Theravada, Mahayana, and Vajrayana. You will see some teachings, some texts, from all three. But the roots are the same. When we look around us at the world today, we see that the teachings are still very useful.'

'What about Buddhism in Cambodia today? You have lost so many monks and nuns.'

'We must take one step at a time, one breath at a time.'

Some westerners find the teachings of Buddhism full of fatalism; the focus on suffering, and the acceptance of suffering, too passive or too likely to lead to tolerance of the intolerable. If you hear only the first (life is suffering) or second (the cause of suffering is attachment) of the four noble truths, this is understandable. But Buddhism goes two steps further. The third truth is the remedy for suffering (mindfulness, meditation, practice). And the fourth is of the reality of liberation. In a place like Cambodia today, in dealing with a social and medical disaster like AIDS, it is not hard to see suffering. What empowers and enlivens is being reminded by teachers like Maha Ghosananda that there is a way out.[4] The Buddha's last words say this with enlightened simplicity: *Work out your own salvation with diligence.*

Notes

1. Cambodia's UN-monitored elections were won by the royalist FUNCIN-PEC Party under the leadership of Prince Ranariddh, a son of Prince Norodom Sihanouk. However, the defeated CPP (Cambodian People's Party) under Hun Sen, the leader supported by Vietnam after the fall of the Khmer Rouge in 1978, demanded to be included in the ruling coalition. Hun Sen, a former Khmer Rouge leader himself, had the largest army in Cambodia at the time, and threatened a return to war if he was not given power. The UN capitulated to this demand in an effort to avoid further fighting. The Cambodian people were thus, once again, denied their choice of government. Ranariddh is officially First Prime Minister and Hun Sen the Second, but he is widely regarded as the real power in Cambodia.

2. While this book was in press, Cambodia's unstable coalition came to a violent end with the *coup d'état* of Hun Sen in June 1997. First Prime Minister Ranariddh went into exile, and his forces began fighting Hun Sen's in western Cambodia, threatening a return to all-out civil war. The agony of the Khmer people continues.

3. Personal communication, *Cambodian Women's Development Association*.

4. In July 1997, four weeks after Hun Sen's violent *coup*, Maha Ghosananda led a peace march through the streets of Phnom Penh to encourage the country's leaders to resolve their political differences without resorting to violence. Reuters estimated that perhaps 1,300 people, led by hundreds of Buddhist monks and nuns, braved the guns to walk with Maha in support of peace.

5. Laos: travels in the Cold War

The health status of the people of Laos is poorly documented and little understood. The Lao People's Democratic Republic remains a closed state, her bamboo curtain still drawn. There is little on Laos in the medical literature, and the Lao lay media are limited and heavily censored. Government publications are fairly crude propaganda and of uncertain credibility. Rural areas – most of the country is rural – are beyond the reach of researchers and the press, and in some areas even of the government. There are few roads, and there has never been a yard of rail. After the region-wide floods of 1994 there were persistent rumors of severe rice shortages, even of famine, in several parts of Laos; these reports were neither confirmed nor denied. In 1995 there were reports of a major outbreak of cholera in several flooded provinces; these reports also were neither confirmed nor denied. Parts of Laos are so uncharted that in 1995 a new ethnic group was discovered in the mountains, a people who had managed to miss both the French colonial period and the nine-year war with the Americans. Laos is not on the information highway. It is a place to which you have to *go*.

One large survey of HIV has been reported from Laos. This was a study among 9,449 persons resident in Vientiane, the capital, between January 1990 and April 1993. The survey was a collaboration between the Hôpital Mahosot, Vientiane, and the Hôpital Cochin, Paris. They found only a few cases: 18 were confirmed out of the whole sample, about 0.2%, roughly one in five hundred persons. The majority of infected persons, 13 of the 18, were women aged 15–29. Twelve of these young women had worked as sex workers in either China or Thailand prior to testing HIV-positive. Most of the tests (5,176) done in this survey were among blood donors. Tellingly, none were HIV-infected (95% of these donors were men.) By 1993, one Lao had officially died of AIDS.

Based on this evidence, if we take it as reliable, we can say several things about HIV in the Lao PDR as of 1993. Compared to its neighbors (Laos has borders with Thailand, Burma, Cambodia, Vietnam, and China) there wasn't much. The finding in blood donors is encouraging; this is a large sample and it suggests little spread in the general population. What HIV cases there were turned up among Lao women and girls who had worked in neighboring countries' sex industries; these were more likely to have been imported cases than evidence of local spread.

But there are problems with these findings. Vientiane is not Laos. This was an urban sample in an overwhelmingly rural country. The border regions with Burma (the Shan state) and with Yunnan, are not represented at all, and these areas certainly have the potential for being key points of HIV introduction and spread. And the data stop in 1993. If the Thai surveillance had stopped in 1987 we might also think of Thailand as a country with little cause for concern. The introduction to the Mahosot–Cochin study bears some scrutiny.

HIV infection in Lao Republic

B.C. Prasongsith, P. Blanche, K. Phouvang, S. Insisiengmay, V. Rajpho, D. Sicard.

A rising incidence of human immunodeficiency virus (HIV) infection has been reported in Thailand and to a lesser extent in Southern China. The Lao People's Democratic Republic (Lao PDR) is located in the heart of the Indochinese peninsula, between Burma and China to the north, Cambodia to the south, Vietnam to the east, and Thailand to the west. The opening of the Lao economy, the building of routes and the completion of the Mekong River bridge between Thailand and Lao PDR could lead to an increase in the incidence of HIV infection. Lao PDR is 80% mountainous, with a low density of population (17/km^2), mostly rural, so that a national sero-survey is difficult to organize.

This introduction nicely shapes what could be called the Lao dilemma. The heart of Indochina is land-locked, sparsely populated and poor. But it is surrounded by crowded countries in dynamic periods of growth and change, with booming economies and increasingly serious social problems. Laos's neighbors want Laos open. They want hydroelectric power from its mountain rivers, they want its timber, they want trade on the Mekong River and they want roads. As it stands, Laos's continued self-imposed isolation blocks road or rail connections between Thailand and China, between Thailand and Vietnam, and between northern Thailand, north-western Laos, the Shan states of Burma, and Yunnan, the 'Golden Quadrangle' economic and travel zone that all the other countries agree could make them richer if Laos would only comply. So far, the Party has resisted.

The Thai–Lao Friendship Bridge mentioned by the Mahosot–Cochin researchers was built with Australian development funds. It officially opened in 1994, connecting Vientiane with Nong Khai, in Thailand's northeast. Ordinary Laotians are not allowed to cross it without special permission, because of government concerns over 'traffic safety.' Once across, they are usually allowed only 3 days in Thailand, and are not allowed to leave Nong Khai province. Travel is tightly controlled by the Politburo of elderly communist generals (thought to be 7 men) who have ruled since 1975.

HIV is just one of a list of threats that Laotians perceive will come with openness and travel. The Party, a Lao contact suggested, is more afraid of ideas and information than viruses. The leadership may have other worries as well. Increasing openness might reveal the extent to which their aged oligarchy is supported by opium revenues. Laos is number two, after Burma, in world opium and heroin production. Not surprisingly, the Lao PDR was the first government in the world to recognize the SLORC, three weeks after the 1988 crackdown in Burma. Ties are close. Heroin is, with hydroelectric power, timber, and a small coffee crop, the only significant foreign-income earner the country has.

The heroin business also involves the Lao leadership's unresolved conflicts with the nation's traditional opium growers, the Hmong and Yao ethnic nationalities. These peoples began opium cultivation to pay the head tax demanded by France during the colonial period. They fought for the French, and subsequently the Americans, during the Indochinese wars; these loyalties led to severe reprisals by the communists once they took power. Some estimates are that a quarter of the Hmong population, some 250,000 people, were killed, and another 200,000 driven into exile, by the Pathet Lao. Many of these refugees found shelter in Thailand and, eventually, in the US. Those that did not make it out of the Thai refugee camps were still there in 1993. The repatriation of these remaining Hmong refugees back to

Laos is one of the last acts of the Vietnam era passion play. It was almost completed in 1996, but tensions still run high. There have been rumors of a resurgent Hmong resistance to the Lao regime, rumors that again have been difficult to verify or discount. What is happening in the highlands is as hidden as the roadless ranges themselves.

How vulnerable is Laos to HIV? Between 1994 and 1996 I made three trips there in an attempt to answer this question, to study this enigmatic place in the 'heart of Indochina'. The first was a short and unproductive trip to Vientiane. The second a longer journey, overland and by boat, down the Mekong to Luang Prabang, the old capital. The third, a visit to the most heavily bombarded place on earth, the Plain of Jars, and from there north, to poppy growing areas near the border with Vietnam, what used to be called the Ho Chi Minh trail.

Vientiane

Arriving in Vientiane from Chiang Mai is like stepping off a flight from JFK into a wide Montana afternoon. The skies are astonishing. The afternoon I landed it was a high clear blue with puffy banks of cumulus overhead. There was a band of soft river light to the south, over the Mekong, vertical rain falling to the far north, a fierce brilliant sun just off-center to the west. Such skies are history in Chiang Mai, where bands the color of nicotine hang perennially over the valley, and even the bluest reaches are dull with dust and lead.

Vientiane is slow. What little traffic there is glides over the rutted roads with a cadence more like boating than driving. It's striking after frenetic Thai traffic. The population was supposed to be 493,505 in 1995, but it feels more like one-tenth of that. The city sits beside a wide stretch of the Mekong. Where the flood waters have receded, locals have planted vegetable patches in the river bed, giving the city a scraggy backdrop of corn tassels. The feel is much more of a provincial town than a city, a town with several grandiose monuments which suggest not so much that this is a capital city, but that the state they are meant to represent is something of a historical fiction, and an unconvincing one. There is the Lao version of the Arc de Triomphe, rising high above a traffic circle and facing the Presidential Palace in a dramatic layout that is pure Paris. Instead of power, it suggests a very threadbare colonial vision of what might have been.

The same can be said of the enormous and criminally ugly constructions of the Soviets. Peeling and cracking, they suggest less the fraternity of a socialist international than another vision of Laos which contrasts jarringly with the actual town, a place of low, ramshackle houses, banana trees growing out of pavements, kids and chickens and dogs padding about in the dust.

There is no daily newspaper, but the *Bangkok Post* is available intermittently. There is a weekly *Vientiane Times* in English, fascinating reading from a cultural, if not a news, standpoint. What educated Laotians actually use for news is a mimeographed daily 'fact sheet' which has telegraphic shorts on international matters extracted from the Chinese *Xinhua* news service, as well as bulletins from the Lao Government. It is actually written in decent English, and, surprisingly, reported news both of rice shortages in Luang Prabang province and of a cholera outbreak north of Vientiane.

I will spare you the frustrations of trying to arrange meetings in Vientiane. A low-level official chuckled at my attempts and told me that 'Lao PDR' stands for Laos Please Don't Rush. Expatriates have it as Lao Per Diem Required – if you don't pay officials to attend meetings, the doughnuts and coffee are all yours.

The one, not unqualified, success of this trip was a journey inland to one of the large dams built to harness Laos's hydroelectric power. We made the journey inland in a huge Chinese flatbed truck. This took us north of Vientiane and up toward the highlands. There were very few other vehicles on the road once we left the city (although we still managed to collide with one, a Soviet Laika sedan that our Chinese charger crunched with impunity). The only significant traffic was of logging trucks, a steady stream of them bearing the trunks of immense trees heading north to China, whose booming economy is starved for hardwoods, long a symbol of wealth to the Chinese. We never made it to the dam, as our vehicle lost several gears, and ceased to be able to negotiate the steeply graded roads. But we did get fairly far into the countryside, and it is here that the country reveals something more of itself.

Rural Laos is, if anything, slower than Vientiane. It is very much a traditional subsistence economy of small scattered towns and villages. There is little evidence of trade, or of any surpluses with which to trade. With the exception of saw mills cutting timber for the trucks, there is not much sign of anything like industry. Where the land is flat and has enough water, it is paddy country. But that year's monsoon had been heavy and much of the lowland was still flooded.

The countryside is an ethnic patchwork as complex as the paddy plots. Each village seems ethnically distinct from the next; beside a Hmong community is a Tai Dam one, then a Lao, then a Yao, then perhaps another Tai Dam, or subgroup of Laos. What they have in common is poverty. Most houses are simple shacks without running water or electricity. Toilets are outdoor latrines, often built over running streams. Where there are sewage systems (we saw a few in the larger towns) these are raw open drains. It's not hard to see why cholera remains such a problem here. The men thigh deep in the paddy are also vulnerable to the flukes and parasites so common in these regions. Children with kwashiorkor were common in some villages, especially the Hmong ones, where most of the younger kids we saw were malnourished.

Luang Prabang

Luang Prabang is the old capital of Laos, the royal city of the Lao Kingdom in earlier times. It is on the Mekong, like Vientiane, but on a section of the river that cuts deep into the country, and is ringed by mountains. While no longer a commercial center, it retains its place as the gem of Lao culture and architecture. In Lao it's usually called *Mong Luang*, main city. To get there you can cross Thailand's far north by road, and cross the Mekong where it forms the Thai–Lao border. This takes you to Ban Huai Sai, where you can catch freight boats to Luang Prabang.

Ban Huai Sai looks modern and ugly, but is in fact an old trading town. It was here, in the 18th and 19th centuries, that trading caravans from Yunnan came down from the Silk Road and met the Mekong. They crossed with their goods to Chiang Khong in Thailand, and traded them in Chiang Rai and Chiang Mai. They then crossed back to take the river to the old Lao capital. This ancient route is catching on again. Chinese laborers come down to Ban Huai Sai looking for work in Laos. Goods come up from Chiang Rai, are ferried across, and go either north by road or down the Mekong. The goods include guns, which are sold openly on the streets of Ban Huai Sai, and the chemicals necessary to turn opium into heroin. North of Ban Huai

Sai, it has been reported (but, of course, not confirmed) that there are several large heroin refineries. Shan opium is also reportedly refined in northern Laos. The old Silk Road takes the purified white powder to Kunming, in China. From there it is flown to Shanghai, then Hong Kong, then out to the markets of the West. So this small and seemingly sleepy little river port is one key link in the chain that eventually leads to the agonies of Harlem, Newark, and Watts.

The road north out of Ban Huai Sai, which connects Thailand to southern China, is slated to be a key part of the growth zone of the economic quadrangle. Its development is planned with support from the Asian Development Bank. If this comes to pass, Ban Huai Sai will change radically. How this will affect the heroin trade is yet another unknown. (The idea of the conservative ADB helping to improve the infrastructure for the heroin industry would be amusing if it were not so sad.)

Just after dawn, we climb onto the tin roof of a freight boat. We will sit on this roof for two days. Two days in which we see perhaps 20 villages altogether, one small market town, and miles and miles of dense green mountain forest.

Several of the villages we pass are Hmong. These are new villages, though because they're bamboo and thatch, they look as old as any of the other river-bank hamlets. This area is not traditional Hmong land. They were always mountain farmers, not river-folk. But the deep mistrust of the Hmong for the government in power has kept them close to Thailand, where the refugee camps are only a few hours by boat. And, like the Khmer refugees, many Hmong cannot go home owing to land-mines and unexploded 'ordnance'.

The river is swollen. I sit with the captain for a few hours to avoid the sun. We are carrying asbestos roof tiles to Luang Prabang, and the barge is overloaded. The wheel he turns is rigged to iron chains that run on each side of the 30-foot craft, and turn the rudder at its end. Because of the weight and length of the barge, he has to anticipate a wide backswing, and glide the boat over rapids as its stern trails now wide to the left, now too far to the right. The chains are responsive to the wheel, but the boat is not easily handled, and he is in constant motion, eyes on the rocks, the currents, the way ahead. In two days of constant travel he never comes close to a rock, never comes near a spill over the rapids, never slows down. Under-development develops people, if nothing else.

The country is spectacular. The mountains are dense and closely packed, dropping steeply to the river with dark granite walls. Everything is green after the rains. There is very little sign of people here. Every few kilometers you see what looks like the remains of a field, some scattered plantings of corn or banana. In some stretches we move for several hours without seeing a soul.

When we stop for the night, the captain invites us to drink shots of the local moonshine, called Lao Lao. Made from rice, it has a faint taste of licorice, with a hint of gasoline. It comes in a plastic bag, and there is only one glass, filled to the brim and emptied in one fiery gulp. After the third, or fourth, I actually like it, though there is the lingering fear of it being methanol, not ethanol, and waking up permanently blind.

Sitting around the fire after dinner, I ask the men if they have heard of AIDS. Yes, they have, they know it's spread by sex, and they know it kills you, but they all agree that it is only in Thailand, not in Laos. I ask the captain if he thinks he is in any danger of becoming infected.'No. Because I don't do anything that would put me in danger. I am married, I stay with my wife. She is very beautiful. And I don't go to brothels, even in Vientiane.'

Dawn, when it finally comes, is damp and chilly. Our captain is up before first light, working the fire. After a sickeningly sweet coffee each, we crawl back onto the boat and huddle on the wet tin roof. If it wasn't hard to get to this place, it wouldn't be what it is. All the comfortable places in this crowded region are packed to the gills.

Another day of green mountains, pink buffaloes, blue kingfishers, and the river twisting and winding its way through gorges, over rapids, into wider, slower stretches. We have cut sharply away from Thailand now, and the river is running almost due east toward the city. There are still only a handful of hamlets and fields cut out of hillsides. The buffaloes must be inbred: more than half are albinos, pink where caked mud has cracked on their hides, with milky white muzzles and dull gray eyes.

There is no sign as we approach that the old city is near. There are no outlying towns, no roads, only a few more long-nosed boats, and a handful of barges. The city doesn't actually appear as we come round the last bend. There are just banks coated with garbage, and four or five stairways leading up from the shore. Luang Prabang is a town of about 8,ooo people.

In the afternoon we visit the house of a Lao family who sell old weaving and embroidery, one of the Lao high arts. The woman who runs the business is about 40, a classic beauty: delicate features, wide-set cocoa-brown eyes, and thick, straight black hair to her waist. Her mother joins us, an equally lovely old lady, with the same eyes, and her white locks in a high bun. They were connected to the court in the old days, and have suffered greatly. Their men are gone. Beside the cash register in the shophouse are several photos of their daughter in traditional dress. Another stunning face, and impossibly slender limbs and waist. The mother tells me proudly that her daughter was 'Miss New Year' in the last beauty pageant. A Thai businessman paid a 10,000-Baht bride-price for her and took her to live in Bangkok. They have not seen her since, but are sure that she is alright, for the Thai man was rich. The Thai man told the family that he wanted her for a wife, and I hope that is true, but the likelihood is that she is locked in a brothel or massage parlor somewhere, servicing an endless string of men. There are many versions of this story, and 10,000 Baht (about US$400) is the standard rate for women trafficked into the flesh trade. Wives usually cost more.

The Luang Prabang Provincial Hospital is on the main street in town, ringed by a low stone wall, behind which is a lawn gone to seed. The buildings are one-storey French, circa 1930s, and clearly not renovated since. Rather than go through official channels, which I've been told can take months, I tell a nurse crossing the grass that I need to see a doctor. She leads me into a large empty room, with one desk and two low benches in a corner. A young woman joins us after a few minutes, and this is the doctor. She has a bright open face and a welcoming smile. I give her my card, explain the purpose of my visit, and ask her if she has a few minutes to talk. She speaks Russian (trained in Moscow in Internal Medicine), Lao, a bit of French, and some Thai. I speak Thai, fair French, and understand about half of what is said in Lao. This leads to a word-salad conversation, a tower of Babel for two, but, medicine being medicine, we can passably follow each other. She does not offer her name, or a card, and I sense that I shouldn't push for this.

The hospital has 200 beds, and a staff of 12 medical doctors supported by another 20 or so health aides and nurses. As Laos has no medical school, all the doctors have been trained overseas, the very elderly in France, but since the 1960s in the Soviet world: in the Soviet Union itself, in Cuba, Hungary, and Vietnam. Now that Soviet aid for education has stopped, they are hoping to send the next generation to Thailand, where there is no language barrier, and no long Russian winters.

The single largest problem here is malaria, which is endemic in much of Laos. More than half the in-patients are malaria cases, especially children with cerebral malaria. Many of the current cases have falciparum, the most aggressive of the four malaria parasites. Antibiotic resistance is a major problem. After malaria, tuberculosis is next, then diarrhea, cholera, malnutrition, and accidents, which often lead to infected wounds. As we walk the crowded, dirty wards, it is clear that HIV would be a disaster here. Because people with HIV infection are so susceptible to tuberculosis, and there is already so much TB, an African situation, with both diseases running rampant, could make this place a charnel house.

'Have you seen any HIV cases here? Any clinical AIDS?'

'We don't have resources to test as many people as we should. This we know. We test women from Luang Prabang coming home from working in Thailand, because we know many of them have worked in brothels there. So far we have found only three with HIV. They all came back with money and got married soon after, so we know HIV is here. We don't see many heroin addicts who use needles. Even we can't get enough needles! But I personally am worried because now we have so many Chinese laborers, and laborers coming in from the Shan states. Next year the government wants to have direct air flights from Chiang Mai to Luang Prabang, so we must be prepared. We are surrounded by AIDS countries.'

'Do you think the medical staff here would like to have some training in AIDS control and care?'

'Definitely, yes. There is a lot we don't know. But you will have to speak to the Minister of Health about this, in Vientiane. I will introduce you to his deputy in Luang Prabang.'

'What about prostitution here?'

'We don't really have that, only in Vientiane.'

'I was told there are prostitutes at the R____ hotel, and at the disco.'

'Yes, that is true.'

The head of the Pediatrics department, another woman, was

trained in Havana. I dig up my high school Spanish from somewhere, and we are back to word salad, this time with a salsa twist. She shows me a ward full of children with cerebral malaria, a major cause of death here. There are two little boys, brothers, with their father and grandfather, both boys in deep coma after a three-day walk to the hospital. The men are anguished, startled to see a white face, and then hostile when it's clear that I have nothing to offer their dying sons.

The surgery is a part of medical history, with used surgical gloves washed and hung up to dry like hand towels. There is an autoclave, actually working, to sterilize the tools, a donation from the US from before the fall of Saigon. The intensive care unit, such as it is, has no working oxygen, no suction, no ventilators. This is not a place to have a serious illness, and it is the only hospital for hundreds of miles in these rugged mountains.

'What do you do for cases that need oxygen?'

'We try to get them to Vientiane by plane. If they have money, and if we can arrange it, we send them to Udon.' Udon is the Air America base in northern Thailand from which we sent over the payloads dumped on these people for nine long years.

All together I talked with seven physicians, all women. I found out later that they each earn 38,000 Kyip a month, less than US$40. The government prohibits doctors from having private clinics, which is why, I find out later, there are no men left working as physicians – you can't support a family on a physician's wages.

On our way to meet the Deputy Minister of Health, we leave the hospital compound and walk to a small building next to a gas station. The walls are covered with health promotion posters, several of which I recognize as AIDS posters put out by the Thai authorities. A staffer tells us they are in Lao, but the writing is clearly Thai. They show bar-boys dancing in bikinis, and people with horrendous end-stage disease – useless messages here, where HIV will not spread though non-existent male hustlers, or wasted dying bodies, but through healthy looking young men and women, as it has throughout Asia.

'Good morning, I am the deputy here. Ah, you are from Thailand. Interested in AIDS, I see. Of course Thailand has a lot of AIDS. We don't have this problem here. There have been no cases of HIV or AIDS in Luang Prabang. Why not? Well you see, we do not have any drug users here, and we do not have prostitution. Also, Lao people are not involved in this homosexuality. So we really have no way for HIV to spread here.'

The young lady doctor spoke up, and I liked her hugely for her courage.

'We have had three cases already, sir.'

'Three, I thought it was only two. Yes, well, one has gone back to Thailand already for treatment.'

'We were hoping to do an HIV course for the medical staff here. Do you think the Ministry would support this idea?'

'Oh yes, why not, we are very open to improving our capabilities. Always open.'

'Could I ask you about drug use? Do you see this as a problem in Laos?'

'It is a problem in every country, isn't it? But it is much less common now than in the past. Our people are very simple, you understand. And we have taken steps.'

'Steps?'

'When the Americans were here, Laos was full of these drugs. Now you see, it is only some of the older people, tribal people. They think of opium as a medicine. This is changing, but it is slow. Perhaps you should speak to my superior. He can tell you more.' And then, at last, a name: the Minister of Health for the Lao PDR, and his address. We are far from the communist mainstream here, but the archetype, the party functionary toeing the line, is alive and well in Luang Prabang.

The Plain of Jars

The Plain of Jars (Plain des Jarres – PDJ to war buffs) was one of the most heavily contested theaters of the secret war in Laos. The US had no ground troops there, just CIA operatives and the Hmong. The North Vietnamese had perhaps 70,000 troops on the high plateaus around Xiang Khoang, the only major town on the PDJ. The US strategy was to bombard the communists by air, waging an aerial campaign against the Ho Chi Minh trail without using US ground troops. This went on for nine years and was a manifest failure. When the US had had enough of bombing and went home, the Hmong were swiftly defeated, and the Plain of Jars fell under Vietnam's control. The people of Xiang Khoang had lost their city, their countryside, and, in many cases, their lives. The region today is desperately poor. The US mission was in one sense a success: we wanted 'to bomb them into the stone age', and just about did.

There was no plane available on the day we wanted to go to the PDJ, but an old Soviet transport helicopter had been pulled out of storage from somewhere. The door didn't exactly shut, which meant the Lao flight attendant spent the entire ride holding on to it. The view of the mountains was especially nice through the seams in the chopper floor.

Once airborne you pass quickly out of the settled plain around Vientiane. For many miles there is nothing below but green mountains, snaky rivers cutting through unfarmed valley floors, and high stone ridges bare of trees. The country dries out as you head north; the forests are replaced first by low scrub, then by bare earth studded with rock. About fifty miles from the PDJ the craters begin to appear. It is impossible to see now what was being bombed. Many high brown ridges, completely devoid of green, are pocked and punched and bitten with craters. What had been there? Villages? Troops dug into bunkers? Cattle grazing? Were there forests? Was this landscape always lifeless, or did we do that? Nearer to Xiang Khoang the craters are virtually everywhere. It looks like smallpox, on land instead of skin. There are huge circular chunks missing from the scattered fields, from the sides of hills, gouged out of the flat spaces. The old city of Xiang Khoang, capital of an ancient and little documented Lao–Thai kingdom, was bombed into oblivion. Erased. The new town, which we are just about to enter, looks bleak from the sky. Everything standing is post-1975. There is no evidence, from the air, of the famous jars.

After a soft slow landing we climb out of the helicopter into a blast of frigid, dusty wind. The plain around us is brown, bleak, empty, more like Mongolia than Southeast Asia. The arrivals building is a rattan-walled shack. We get our police stamp, and we meet Duang Sai Jai (in English 'to add stars to your heart'). He's a young Lao guide with a jeep and he speaks Thai. After a few minutes of negotiation, we're off.

Driving through this countryside is a lesson in the aftermath of war. The surviving people, in their poverty and ingenuity, have come up with an incredible array of uses for what gets left after nine years of bombardment. Their pig troughs are made of bomb casings; the rice barns are raised off the ground on bomb casings; a farmer's plough uses the base of a tank. Scrap from the war is used to make water pumps, fence posts, and shack foundations. In the end, what fell from the sky was made of metal. It is a pity we didn't just drop real pig troughs.

The jars of the PDJ are a fitting attraction for the place. Cut from solid stone, and varying in length from perhaps four to eight feet, they are, quite simply, giant stone jars. Their meaning is lost, and the culture that generated them is unknown (and given the destruction here is likely to remain so). They sit on the land with their open mouths saying whatever they were meant to say to an uncomprehending audience. So too the bomb craters. What was it for and why was it done? What do they mean now, to the local people? The population of Laos is exceptionally young, the older generation having been greatly reduced in number by years of war. The people of Xiang Khoang are mostly post-war kids. They want to learn English, wear blue jeans, dance in discos, and study abroad. The battles that cost their parents everything have been over for 20 years. Duang Sai Jai would like to go to university. Laos does not have a university. He would like to go to Bangkok (they have better brothels there than in Vientiane, he tells me). But it is 'difficult', he says, as he has no family connections to the leadership. The party is not about to let Duang Sai Jai and his friends travel to the capitalist nation next door. And they are never going to forget the nine years of fire falling, day and night, from a faraway enemy in the skies.

We pass through the town of Ponsavanh on our way to the mountains. The modern town was built by the Soviets, after the US destroyed the original one. The people walking along the cold, dusty road are about as poor as you can get; we pass several kids with the orange hair of kwashiorkor, little girls carrying enormous bushels of sticks, gaunt old men on Chinese bicycles, hatless and gloveless in the bitter air. We stop in the market to get some water for a three-hour drive north. There are some mealy cabbages and turnips, some wilted lettuces, and little else. One Khmu tribal woman is selling three freshly killed porcupines. She sits before the fat rodents laid out on a board, methodically plucking quills from their skins with a short knife. Another woman, a blue Hmong, has a pair of grey-green magpies for sale. They've been snared, and their beautiful plumage is intact. It is a species I have never seen before, with a long, curved vermilion bill, white eye patches, and the distinctive long banded tail feathers of the family. Alive, they would be worth a fortune, by Lao standards, on the illegal bird market. Here, they are being sold for meat.

There is only one road going north out of Ponsavanh. You could take it to China if there was a border crossing at its end, but apparently there isn't. The border with Vietnam is about 40 kilometers east of this road, which explains why it was bombed so thoroughly. The land is dry, rocky hills, too steep for rice, but perfect for poppies. Actually the flowers are not in bloom at this time of year; the plants are only about a foot high, and look more like a kind of spinach than those lovely red flowers that carpet the hillsides. The road north has many poppy patches, but Duang Sai Jai insists that the real fields are one ridge over from the road. The fields we do see are mostly tended by little girls. There is little to do but weed at this time of year. It looks like lonely work for children, and there seem to be no adults around, nor even any houses that these small laborers might go home to. I had expected something more sinister than this, but opium is a poor people's crop. The people who grow it see the least fraction of its profits. The money these little girls generate must run to many millions, but it gets laundered and invested in another world, and spent in yet another, the place where the bombs came from.

How vulnerable is Laos? As the sages say, it depends. After these journeys I've come to think the politburo may be right to go slowly in terms of opening Laos to its neighbors, to trade, investment and development. Laos is fragile, its economy marginal, its society still in tatters after years of war. Change will inevitably come to the heart of Indochina, but in what form and on whose terms? Will HIV follow the roads here, as it did into the hinterlands of Africa? It easily could. Are the young generation of Lao women and girls as vulnerable to trafficking as the women of the Khmers, the Shans? Undoubtedly so. Would development lead Laos out of the opium-growing business or push it further down a darker road? Time is still moving at the Laotians' chosen pace, but their neighbors are impatient.

6. Malaysia: ethnicity, activism, and AIDS

The national statistics are not as alarming as in neighboring countries, but we may be deluding ourselves and may actually be facing the iceberg phenomenon, since no detailed epidemiologic study has been conducted on all the high-risk groups in the country.

Professor S.K. Lam, University of Malaya

On World AIDS Day, December 1, 1995, the Malaysian AIDS Council, an umbrella body of 22 AIDS organizations, commemorates those who have died and those still fighting. A memorial service has been organized by Pink Triangle, one of the largest activist groups. The turnout is eclectic. In this ethnically and religiously divided society, the crowd is a rainbow mix of Malays, Chinese, Indians, and expats. There are women covered from crown to toe with only their faces exposed, eating sweets and drinking tea with girls in miniskirts, short spiked hair and pierced noses. A gay couple, both professionals, staff the information booth. One is Malay, the other Chinese. Several gaunt addicts sniffle against a far wall; social activists from Singapore and Indonesia network with diligence; the divine Khartini Salmah, a Malay transgender outreach worker, dishes out plates of food. Khartini also wears a proper ankle-length shift, but she has *big* hair and *serious* nails. There's a dance performance, several dramatic monologues, and an interview for the national radio with Winston Chu, a Malaysian person with AIDS (PWA) who tells his story with heart-wrenching honesty.

Marina Mahathir is among the first to arrive and the last to leave. She is the chairwoman of the AIDS council, a key fundraiser and organizer. She is also the daughter of the country's long-serving Prime Minister, Dato Dr Muhammad Mahathir, head of the United Malay National Organization (UMNO), the party that has ruled

Malaysia for nearly two decades. Marina is arguably the most prominent woman of her generation in the country, but she is no figurehead here; these are her friends. Her classy, natural presence draws the media and inhibits the authorities, a happy conjunction.

This gathering, in Southeast Asia at least, could only be happening in Kuala Lumpur (KL). The language is KL English, swift, articulate, and spicy with other tongues. Most of the organizations represented here are service groups, but many are also activist in orientation. The language and symbols in the room, and on people's clothes, are instantly recognizable as part of the international AIDS movement: pink triangles, rainbow flags, the quilt display, red ribbons on lapels, 'silence = death' and 'action = life', ACT UP, Fight Back, Fight AIDS. Many of the people at the memorial service are friends. After places like Burma and Cambodia, it is a great joy to be able to speak freely, to feel understood, to be with gay men who have been part of the world I come from. These are people who can visit Thailand with real passports, unlike Burmese friends; people who can communicate via e-mail.

The same evening, there's a series of one-act plays commissioned from young local writers. It is called 'Talking AIDS'. Each of the short pieces deals with an aspect of the epidemic in Malaysia. It's a pleasure to hear theater in English, to see Malaysian responses and hear Malaysian ideas in the context of a theatrical tradition that's immediately accessible. Some of the plays are pointedly explicit. In the first, a young woman who's had casual sex after a drunken evening takes the audience through a miserable morning-after anxiety attack. In another, a young rough talks on the phone with one of his buddies – a whoring buddy, who's just been diagnosed. One of the best, written by a Pink Triangle member, is the monologue of a public health official, a conservative Muslim, remembering one of her first cases of AIDS, a young gay man who taught her something about, of all things, love. It is a surprisingly sophisticated, complex portrayal; I had expected a lampoon. But this is the Kuala Lumpur of the new Malaysians, and they are *with it*.

They are not, however, in power; UMNO is, and UMNO is defined by single-party rule, a policy of 'positive discrimination' to support the Muslim majority against the economic clout of the Chinese, strict media censorship, and little or no tolerance of political opposition. Compare the KL daily newspapers to the *Bangkok Post* or

The Nation and you know instantly that the Malaysian print media are only a cut above the unspeakable *New Light of Myanmar* or *The China People's Daily*, full of smiling ministers kissing babies, human interest stories on the virtues of tradition, pages of sports, and advertisements for luxury automobiles. All of which serves to make Malaysia a country of paradoxes, contradictions, and jarringly different official and unofficial versions of events.

The country has done well in development terms; its economic growth has been no less rapid than Thailand's, but investments have been much more evenly distributed. While Thailand has joined the extreme economies of Latin America in terms of iniquitous wealth distribution (it is now one of the world's ten worst countries in terms of the gap between haves and have-nots), Malaysia has steadily raised the living standards of the poor through education and targeted development. The result is an impressively prosperous society, and one where economic opportunity has helped to defuse potent ethnic hostilities, as well as the potential rise of militant Islamic movements. Kuala Lumpur is by far the best managed and most habitable capital city in Southeast Asia. Things work: the roads are a pleasure to drive; the city is full of greenery; the shops are crammed. The recently completed National Mosque is both modern and Islamic: sweeping, harmonious, crisp white lines.

This is not to say that the politics of ethnicity and faith have been resolved, or are anywhere close to declining in importance. The population is approaching 20 million people, and is officially 60% Malay (all Muslim, by UMNO definition), 25% Chinese (Buddhist, Christian, and Confucian), 10% Indian (Hindu and Christian), and perhaps 1–2% indigenous and tribal minorities (Animist, Christian, and Muslim). Religion and ethnicity in Malaysia are not just about food preferences and dress. There are government bank loans reserved for Malays; parts of Kuala Lumpur are 'reserved' for Malay ownership; university entrance exams have different admission criteria for different ethnic groups; the Malay language is heavily promoted. All ethnic Malays are officially Muslims, ensuring a majority Islamic population, at least on paper. There is freedom of worship for all groups, but the UMNO is in firm control of the government, and its policies are true to its name: Malay nationalist. This is a country where race, identity, and religion count in almost every facet of public life. And there is some evidence to suggest that ethnicity may be playing a key role in the distribution of HIV subtypes in Malaysia as well, as we shall see.

The government, military, police, and a considerable bulk of the civil service are Malay, and thus Muslim-dominated. The Chinese are the economic power in the country – bankers, industrialists, developers – and they also dominate the professions, academic life, and medicine. The Indians are too few to dominate any sector, but are active in the professions, trade, and small businesses. There is also a considerable population of illegal workers and migrants: perhaps 200,000 Indonesians and 50,000 Burmese. These are the menial and day laborers, loggers, agricultural workers, servants, and the underclass. There is a Thai population here as well, not large, and not very visible, unless you look at HIV cases – many are Thai women working in swanky 'health clubs' and 'fitness centers' that double as discreet sex venues. This reality, however, is as covert in Kuala Lumpur as it is open in Phnom Penh or Bangkok. Malaysia has many faces. The one UMNO would like the world to see does not include prostitution, or heterosexual promiscuity, or homosexuality. Malaysia's policy on drug use is another matter.

A hard line on drug use is very much a part of the country's identity. As you land on Malaysian soil, the pilot of your aircraft calmly announces, 'Welcome to the Islamic Republic of Malaysia. We have a mandatory death sentence for narcotics trafficking.' And they use it. When I met with the head of Malaysia's national drug enforcement agency (a Malay, one should probably specify here), he showed me the numbers of traffickers hanged, annually, over the past decade. The numbers seemed steady throughout the period, between 175 and 250 per year. I pointed out that if capital punishment were meant as a deterrent, it seemed not to be working. Shouldn't the numbers fall over time? 'Profit, you see. It's just so profitable.' Indeed. But one might add that the mules who carry drugs are mostly 'little people' in desperate need of cash. Hanging them might have little effect on the drug trade.

'Yes. We know this. But we feel very strongly about drug use here.'

'Could needle exchange be used in Malaysia to reduce the spread of HIV among addicts?'

'Yes. But *we* cannot do it. That is for NGOs. As a government body we must enforce the rules that support our national beliefs.'

The system is nothing if not thorough. Police have the right to screen anyone they suspect of drug use with a urine test. Urine is screened for all other routine arrests as well. If the test is positive, you get a mandatory blood test. If that confirms drug use, you get 18–24 months' mandatory incarceration in a drug treatment center. The 'treatment' is cold turkey, as in Burma; no drugs are used to medicate for withdrawal. Does it work? The drug program director said that, unfortunately, many of the admissions were repeat offenders; some had been in and out of treatment three or four times. The failure rate is about 65%, and half the yearly arrests are re-arrests. (These figures do not include the many Malaysian addicts who cross the border into Thailand, where drug detoxification is free, voluntary, lasts three weeks, and includes a methadone taper to get you through withdrawal. About half the patients treated each year at the Thai government treatment center near the border are Malaysians.)

All persons found to have positive tests for drug use (opiates, marijuana, and amphetamines) are also screened for HIV. HIV-infected addicts are segregated in the drug treatment centers, to 'protect' the other addicts from HIV infection. Condoms are not distributed in these centers, although condom use has been discussed recently (after proposals from AIDS activist groups demanding that men in detention be allowed to protect themselves). The HIV rate among arrested addicts is a steady 15%, and has been stable for several years. This is much lower than Thailand, and very much lower than Burma, and probably reflects the greater availability of needles and the higher educational level of Malaysian addicts. This is a somewhat different population of users than in other settings: the majority are employed at the time of arrest, and many are working- or middle-class. Addicts are found among all ethnic groups, though the majority are young Malay men. And that is part of the anxiety.

Death sentences for traffickers, mandatory screening for drug use, mandatory two year incarcerations: put this together and you have a society seriously committed to drug control. It has been this commitment that has shaped Malaysia's response to AIDS.

'Seek and ye shall find' is a motto in public health. If you screen all of one group for a disease, and do not systematically screen others, you will find the problem where you have looked for it. This is a fair representation of the HIV situation in Malaysia. The first reported case was detected in 1986. Most of the early cases occurred among recipients of imported blood products (hemophiliacs) who were systematically screened, homosexual men returning from abroad, and injecting drug users (IDU). By December 1995, the time of the World AIDS Day celebration in Kuala Lumpur, 14,418 cases of HIV infection had been reported, and 331 cases of AIDS. The majority of these reported cases, 77%, were among addicts. But the great majority of HIV tests had been done on addicts. The prevalence of HIV in the general population, based largely on the screening among addicts, was estimated at 0.02/100,000 in 1987, and had risen to 17.5/100,000 by 1995. That is the official story. (The equivalent 1995 figure for Thailand would be 2,100/100,000 persons, to give some perspective, though the Thai data are considerably more reliable.)

However, it is widely acknowledged that there is significant under-reporting of both HIV infections and AIDS cases and deaths. The Ministry of Health estimates that by 1995 there were probably at least 30,000–40,000 HIV-infected persons in Malaysia. Other estimates have been higher, including one of up to 100,000 HIV-infected persons by 1995. These numbers would still differ considerably from Thailand, where after a similar initial epidemic among IDU, the explosive phase was of spread largely through sexual transmission. Perhaps it is true that there is little sexual risk in Malaysia, and that HIV will remain confined to the country's drug users. But perhaps not. Without systematic studies among people at sexual risk – pregnant women, people attending STD clinics, gay men – it will be impossible to know. Such studies are problematic in UMNO's Malaysia. This is an Islamic society still, and there is considerable discomfort with the idea of heterosexual spread of HIV.

Just how uncomfortable was made clear to me in an interview with the Director of the Malaysian National AIDS Program, Dr Harrison Aziza. She told me in no uncertain terms that promotion of condom use was not acceptable in Malaysian society, that HIV vaccines were also unacceptable, and that safer-sex education was definitely not on the national agenda. When I asked what might be acceptable, she warmed:

'Malaysia is leading the way with education. We are not promoting "safe sex", but "right sex". "Right sex" is sexuality in the context of monogamous marriage. We are teaching these values, Islamic family values, to our school children. This is societal prevention for HIV and other STDs. We believe that not only will this prevent HIV, it will also prevent all the other social problems associated with pre-marital sex, extra-marital sex, and other unacceptable sexual behaviors. This is our policy, and we are aware that it is not a Western one. But we are a traditional society, and we have the right to choose our approach to these problems. The West has not done so well with its approaches, so why should we copy them?'

It should be mentioned that Dr Aziza has a Master's degree in public health from Johns Hopkins University and lived, for a time, in Baltimore, a city with very high pregnancy rates in the public schools, a chronic and widespread heroin problem, a homicide rate perhaps ten times that of Kuala Lumpur, and a good many more HIV-infected persons than she currently has to deal with. It is easy to be critical of the UMNO approach. It is much harder to admit the awful shortfalls of our own attempts to manage social problems, unsafe sex among the young, and drug use. The US currently has about 40,000 new HIV infections each year, more than in all of Malaysia since the epidemic began.

'Do you think there's a place for safer-sex education among people already engaged in sex? I mean sex workers and gay men, for example.'

'Yes, of course. But *we* cannot do it. That is what NGOs are for, to deal with these marginalized groups. Our concern is with the future generation. And after all, these groups are very small in our country.'

Fair enough, I thought as I left her. She had several points. But if HIV was already spreading among adults, would Islamic education of schoolchildren not be too late to stem the tide? Education for schoolchildren could take years to bear fruit, assuming it worked at all. What I did not say, since I was a guest in her office and had not been invited to criticize her proposals, was that there was already a significant body of evidence to suggest that sexual risks in Malaysia were much more common than the government was ready to admit.

The Ministry of Health collaborated with the World Health Organization in 1992 in a large survey of the health and behavior of Malaysian adults. This study was the first of its kind in the country, and sought to measure potential vulnerability to sexual spread of HIV. A total of 2,270 adults were interviewed regarding their sexual histories. The majority of married adults, 55%, reported having had sex before marriage, and 29% had between 2 and 10 lifetime sexual partners, which, if you're familiar with these numbers in other cultures and settings, is impressive. How many had had only one sex partner in their lives? Just 38%. Of men who reported ever having had sex, 33% said they had had 'casual' sex in the past year. In addition, 11% of married men reported extra-marital, casual sex in the past year. Not Sodom and Gomorrah, but not Iran either. In fact, these rates of sexual activity are not very different from reports of Thai behavior, which is why they caused a considerable stir in Malaysian medical circles. Malays tend to see the Thais as licentious and permissive Buddhists. By comparison, their own culture is supposed to be much more disciplined and sexually continent. The WHO survey findings suggest that despite the rhetoric, sexual behavior in the general population of both countries is not as different as the bodies politic would prefer. These findings, it must be said, have not been used to guide government HIV-prevention programs in Malaysia. It may also be true that much of the sex reported in the 1992 study did not actually take place in Malaysia.

Malaysians are the largest single group of visitors to Thailand, at over a million per year, according to TAT, the Tourism Authority of Thailand. There is discreet prostitution in Kuala Lumpur's red light district, but for many Malaysians Thailand's border to the north offers close and much safer venues for sexual services than their home communities. The Thai border provinces of Hat Yai, Yala, and Songkhla have developed a thriving commercial sex industry geared to these Malaysian (and Singaporean) visitors. This includes not only straight sex but also gay prostitution, live sex shows, erotic shops, the usual tacky trappings of commercial sex in Asia. A 1993 study of 503 sex workers in Thailand working near the Malaysian border found that 97% of their clients were non-Thai nationals, the majority being Malaysians and Singaporeans. These border area sex workers reported that Malaysian men were much more likely to request sex without condoms than were Thai men. Thai men have been bombarded with safer-sex messages, Malaysians have not. There could be cultural differences at work here as well, but again, little is known about the attitudes of Malaysian men to condom use.

The Isthmus of Kra is a border zone for Malaysia, Thailand, and Burma. All three nations share it, and it was long contested by

England and France. Indeed, the Thais ceded four southern provinces on the isthmus to Britain in the 19th century, and these now make up Malaysia's four northernmost states. The Burmese port of Mergui on the isthmus was also Thai until the 19th century. What has now developed is a new 'triangle trade'. The cross-border sex purchasers are Malaysians, the businesses are owned and run by Thais, and the sex workers are overwhelmingly Burmese women and girls, trafficked from Burma's zones of civil war and poverty. Conditions are appalling. Many of the women are debt-bonded slaves. This may not be what ASEAN has in mind when its foreign ministers talk about 'regional initiatives', but it is a reality, fueled by Malaysia's puritanism, Burma's hungers, and Thailand's expertise in offering tourists what they want but wouldn't dare purchase at home.

This triangle has already produced an AIDS disaster for Thailand and Burma, and is likely to do so for Malaysia as well. On the Burmese side, the isthmus port of Kawthaung reported the highest rates of HIV among men attending STD clinics of any region in Burma: over 30% in 1995. The Thai province with the highest rates of HIV in the general population, after those in the far north of the country, is Ranong, at the northern edge of this southern border zone. It would be a miracle if HIV did not cause similar problems in Malaysia, especially given the reluctance of Malay men to wear condoms. Until the Malays begin to screen the general population, however, this will remain unknown.

One piece of this puzzle has recently come to light, through an unexpected set of findings. Because HIV has multiple subtypes, finding different subtypes in different groups in a population can tell us something about how HIV is spreading. The classic example is again Thailand, where the B subtype of HIV, the predominant virus in the West in both gay men and drug users, accounted for the majority of infections among Thai drug users. In contrast, the explosive spread of HIV among sex workers was largely due to subtype E, suggesting that there was not one epidemic in the country, but two, and that they were not tightly linked, at least initially. Until recently, the HIV subtypes circulating in Malaysia were little studied. On two trips to Kuala Lumpur, however, we were given serum samples from the country's blood banks, STD clinics, sex worker clinics, hospitals, and drug treatment centers – about 90 specimens in all. The Walter Reed group studied these for subtype variation, and a fascinating picture quickly emerged. There were again the same two subtypes as in Thailand, but they seemed to cluster not only by risk group (B was more common among drug users, E among those infected sexually and among sex workers) but also by ethnic group. The Indians (all men) had only B, the Malays had an equal mix of B and E, and the ethnic Chinese and Thais had mostly E. Disturbingly for the Malaysians who would resist such findings, about 40% overall were not drug users, and about 10% of subjects were infected prostitutes working in KL itself. This is a small study, but it is none the less a warning; sexual spread of subtype E in Malaysia looks very much as in Thailand. Drug use is not the only issue for Malaysia, however limited the information on heterosexuals.

A further limitation on understanding HIV/AIDS in Malaysia is the lack of information on the sexual behaviors and risks of men who have sex with men. Despite the efforts of groups like Pink Triangle, sex between consenting adult men is a felony in Malaysia, and heavily stigmatized outside cosmopolitan KL. Like so many former British colonies, Malaysia's laws still specify harsh sentences for the heinous crime of 'buggery', that peculiar anal obsession of the British, who felt the need to criminalize it throughout the world. But we should not (however enjoyable it is to do so) bash Britain too much on this score; some of the Malay states are administered under *Sharia*, Islamic law, in addition to Victorian anal fetishism, and *Sharia* heavily penalizes gays and lesbians. We are talking about stoning here, although this reportedly no longer happens. Such laws and penalties make self-reporting of gay or bisexual risks unlikely. Hence nearly all positive cases not ascribed to drug use are listed as either 'heterosexual' or 'unknown' risk categories. It seems contradictory in a country where AIDS activists are so sophisticated, and urban gays so accepted, that gay sex should still be so criminalized. But Malaysia is much larger than KL. And UMNO is unlikely to adopt policies that would risk the ire of the traditional Muslims. In the US, President Clinton quickly abandoned his support for gay rights out of political expediency. Malaysian gays are fed to the same lions, to keep them busy, and from turning on their keepers.

This confusion over risks is not limited to gays. All addicts here are assumed to be sexless, to have no HIV risks other than their drug habits. If true, this would make them unique: in most countries addicts have greater sexual risk for HIV than others, given their poverty and chaotic social lives, and the need to sell sex for drugs. But if you test positive for drugs and for HIV, you got HIV through drug use. Period.

Medicine

The University of Malaya, in Kuala Lumpur, was founded by the British, and it continues to be an English-language institution. The National University, just down the road in the same comfortable suburb of Petaling Jaya, is a Malay institution, founded after independence in the 1960s. They both have undergraduate- and graduate-level programs, medical schools and teaching hospitals. But it is the University of Malaya that has taken the lead in AIDS: this is where the national HIV lab is, and where a good number of Kuala Lumpur's PWAs come for care. It is a beautiful facility. The campus is large and modern, with spacious lecture halls and quality laboratories. Nearly all of the senior medical faculty are ethnic Chinese. Their academic work is world-class, their English flawless, but guarded. The tension between these academics and the government, on whom their budgets depend, is real. A professor of medicine explained how the system of medical admissions works. It is a reasonable example of the kind of accommodations Malaysians are used to making.

Malays are under-represented in the field of medicine, which is currently dominated by Chinese and Indians. Students take their medical-school qualifying exams together, and they are scored identically, but the admission criteria are set later, and these are based on ethnicity. A Chinese student in a given year must score more than 90%, for example, while Malays achieving 80% will be admitted (the exact criteria vary from year to year, and are kept secret). This is done to ensure that the next generation of physicians will be more Malay, less Chinese. Students who still want to be doctors can go overseas, to Australia or the Philippines, for medical education, but they have to do this privately. The system is called 'positive discrimination' and it is really very similar to the US policy of 'affirmative action', although it is aimed at a majority population, not minority ones. Some of the same negative effects are evident. You cannot help but think that the Malay students are there because of their race, not their ability. It also means the the Chinese who do make it are immediately thought to be particularly gifted. Such programs may do much to address imbalances in numbers, but the psychological effects of discrimination, however 'positive', or 'affirmative', are more pernicious.

While the Malaysians may be resistant to investigating some aspects of HIV spread, and while laws against drug use and homosexuality may be harsh, and the medical system discriminatory, there is no question that for a Southeast Asian with HIV infection, Malaysia is a much better place to be than almost anywhere else. The clinics and hospitals are by far the best equipped that I have seen. There is no mistaking the investments that have been made in medical infrastructure, education, and advanced training. The national blood bank is state-of-the-art and superbly run. Malaysia, perhaps alone in the region, has the will and resources to pay for decent HIV/AIDS care.

It may need these resources. If sexual spread follows the Thai pattern, or if it is already under way and simply not yet detected, there could be many more cases than the government has planned for. Given the progressive medical community, Malaysia's committed activists, and the capability already present, there are more reasons to be hopeful than not. And Malaysia does at least offer an example of an ethnically complex post-colonial society committed to co-existence and co-operation. It's *holding*.

7. Vietnam: the Thai model in action

I was gambling and lost money; I fell into despair, losing confidence. Then my friends said to me that drugs can help stop sadness and despair, life will become happy again. At the beginning, I smoked opium just a little. Then I injected it. Gradually, I began using every day and I don't know when I became addicted to drugs. It lasted for over one year then I quit. However, I can't believe that now I have to pay such a high cost.

A former law student and army veteran, now a cyclo driver in Ho Chi Minh City

By February 1995, the Socialist Republic of Vietnam had reported 2,280 cases of HIV infection, 131 cases of AIDS, and 53 AIDS-related deaths. Ho Chi Minh City had reported 1,130 of these cases, Hanoi 5. These numbers, as you have probably surmised, are thought to be gross underestimates; the WHO estimate of probable cases in 1995 was 200,000, about 100 times as high, and this is not disputed in medical circles in Vietnam. The difference is largely attributed to low numbers of persons at risk seeking tests. Still, however small the sample of documented infections has been compared to actual cases, the huge preponderance of HIV in the south, and its rarity in the north, is too sharp a contrast not to contain some truth. Why one city should have more than 200 times as many cases as another is a question that, in Vietnam at least, cannot be answered without turning to history – the wars, Saigon and the Americans, heroin and prostitution, and the complex dual entity that the north and the south of this country make, and sometimes do not make, together.

Heroin is expensive for the Vietnamese. Liquid opium, cruder and weaker, is cheap, though just as addicting. It is thought to be made locally, possibly in Laos, as liquid opium is not a drug available in most places in the world. It is unpopular because its viscosity makes it difficult to inject; its impurities ruin veins. Prolonged use causes deep, difficult-to-heal abscesses in the skin, venous thromboses, and scarring and swelling that can make the arms and legs look strikingly similar to the limbs of those with elephantiasis. Yet liquid opium is the drug of choice in the south.

The country has, according to government estimates, 120,000 addicts who inject liquid opium and/or heroin. Other estimates are as high as 800,000. Most are southerners. The HIV 'take-off' already seen in addicts in Thailand (1988-89) and in Burma (1989-90) came later to Vietnam. Rates among addicts in Ho Chi Minh were about 2% in late 1992; nine months later, 30% of addicts were HIV-positive. Only extensive needle sharing can explain such rapid spread. Needles cost more than drugs in Vietnam. As in Burma, untrained but 'professional' injectors were doing the work of getting the sticky liquid opium into addicts' veins. Needles were, and are, used repeatedly without sterilization. By 1993 another HIV bomb had gone off.

Heroin, as a colleague of mine – herself a recovering addict – told me, is a drug used to treat otherwise unbearable feelings, like emotional pain, hopelessness, rages that cannot be expressed, failures that cannot be rectified, grief that cannot be faced. The deeper you go into the cycle of relief provided by opiates, the deeper the darkness when you can't get a fix. As the cost of the drug eats away at every aspect of an addict's life, the losses mount, the pain increases, and the dose needed to keep the pain at bay increases in turn. All the opiates, including heroin, mimic natural brain compounds called endorphins. Due to this biologic affinity with the human brain, these compounds develop intensely strong physical, as well as emotional, craving. The daily cycle of pain and release, the habit and the physical craving, eventually enslave the addict. Treatment is difficult. Most addicts fail an average of 4–5 attempts before they succeed in quitting. Many do not succeed. One of the effects of opium is to reduce the urge to breathe. (This gives an idea of how deep into the nervous system these agents penetrate; the urge to inhale is as old as the first attempt of life to leave the sea.) When the spiral of use reaches the point where the addict needs huge doses to find relief, the urge to breathe can be suppressed altogether; the quiet death of an overdose is the result, an effect for which morphine has long been used in euthanasia.

Unbearable pain. Rage that can't be expressed. Hopelessness. To have been on any side of the Vietnam conflict has generated these kinds of emotional states in veterans, survivors, refugees, and prisoners of war. Americans who fought here have much higher rates of heroin addiction than the veterans of any other American conflict. Some of this is certainly due to availability, since Vietnam had heroin, and it was practically non-existent for US troops in Korea, or in France in the 1940s. But some of this addiction has also to do with pain. Vietnamese veterans are also susceptible. Imagine having fought on the losing side in this war, and then having to stay. The South Vietnamese Army, the ARVN, was huge. By the end of the American War there were more than 400,000 troops, and enormous numbers of men had already died. Some 110,000 officers and soldiers were arrested after the fall of Saigon, and subjected to re-education. It was not a bloodbath, as some had predicted: 95,000 or more left the camps alive, to return to a life marked by having betrayed the nationalist cause. This cannot have been simple. Ho Chi Minh is a city full of beggars, and not a few of these are disabled and/or drug addicted ex-soldiers who have, for whatever reason, been unable to begin new lives in the Socialist Republic.

You meet many of these men in Ho Chi Minh City (as Saigon became). I was approached several times a day by Vietnamese men looking for Colonel Bob or Captain Pete, their old unit commanders. Here, uniquely in my experience, people wanted to know how old I was, precisely how old. When I told them, they usually smiled diffidently and walked away: too young to have been a part of their war. Many of these men are still waiting for deliverance from the communists. It was a shock to discover how much they missed their American contacts, how much like Americans they were, to hear the accents and phrases of the American south, or midwest, circa 1970: 'Shit yeah, buddy. We'll catch you later.'

But they didn't. For many, heroin was a way to deal with the loss, or the losses. And now it has led, for one-third of the addicts here, to HIV, a much more difficult death than the breathless sleep of an overdose.

Needle exchange, the supply of clean, safe injection equipment, could change this. In one of the painful/beautiful juxtapositions of American–Vietnamese relations, it is a group of American war veterans, also ex-heroin addicts, and many also HIV-infected, who are developing needle-exchange programs in the new Vietnam. The organization is called the National AIDS Brigade, from Boston. Not

all the group are vets, but many are. The exchange is based in Ho
Chi Minh, and it has received support from the government. It was
a health official in Hanoi who told me about the group, and why, in
practical terms, it might work. The advantage of Vietnam's heroin
scene is that you do not have to reach 120,000 (or 800,000) addicts,
educating the several thousand injectors would go a long way. Clean
up their practices, and much of the spread between addicts could be
stopped. Sexual spread is a very different problem, and again, very
different in the south than in the north.

What do the national data show? Here, as written, is the 11
February 1995 report of the National AIDS Control Committee to
Mr Nguyen Khanh, Vice-Premier and Chairman of the Committee:

Analysis of the HIV-positive cases throughout the entire nation

Gender	Number	Percentage
Male	1895	86.1
Female	268	12.2
Not indicated	37	1.7
Total	2200	

Category		
Drug addicts	1719	78.1
Prostitutes	96	4.4
Venereal disease patients	52	2.4
Overseas Vietnamese	21	1.0
Hotel staff	21	1.0
Blood donors	27	1.2
TB patients	25	1.1
Others	63	2.9
Unknown	176	7.9

It is an interesting list. Missing are several groups we would expect
to see, such as homosexual men, pregnant women, military recruits –
populations that are somewhat standard for national statistics on
HIV/AIDS. Present are some unexpected groups, such as 'hotel staff',
and 'overseas Vietnamese'. Presumably 'hotel staff' is a proxy category
for another risk, like having sex with foreigners, or perhaps for gay
men or women selling sex. 'Overseas Vietnamese' is more troubling;
it seems unlikely that Vietnamese resettled in the US or Australia
would reveal their HIV status to the government in Hanoi. A sadder
likelihood is that the last of the 'boat people' era refugees, now being

repatriated to Vietnam, are coming home with HIV after years in camps scattered across Asia. Testing HIV-positive on a health check-up for settlement in the United States, for example, would disqualify an otherwise acceptable refugee. The US does not accept refugees with HIV infection, as any Haitian can tell you.

Several other things are striking about these data: the great preponderance of cases among addicts, a number almost identical to Malaysia; the relatively small number of HIV-positive sex workers, which looks like an underestimate; and the number of cases in blood donors, 1.2% of the total HIV burden. There is only a small number of positive blood donors here, 27 out of 2,200 cases, but this is the only 'general population' group in the national data. It is also striking that the data thus far show an epidemic almost entirely in men. This has been seen in early epidemics of HIV in most settings. Over time, women tend to catch up. In some places, the African epicenter is an example, new cases may be more common in women than in men.

Winds of change

Old Saigon was a sexually permissive place, if only because the massive foreign presence created such a large market for sexual services. The Vietnamese people, however, have traditionally seen their culture as sexually conservative, and communism is always prudish. The actual sexual practices of the general public in Vietnam have been little studied under the communists. After the long years of war, Vietnam went into an extended baby boom; family planning was not given great attention; the population is now over 75 million and expanding rapidly. Vietnam is already one of the most densely populated nations in Asia. The government has had to respond, and has now initiated a two-child-only policy. The government-issue condoms (Vietnam manufactures its own) are called 'Happy Family', and their logo is a family of four: mother, father, one son, one daughter.

But the government is concerned. How much sexual risk is there in Vietnam? How much prostitute use? How many married men have sex outside the family? Their anxiety, which is openly discussed, is that sexual activity in Vietnam may be more like the Thai example than they think, and that a heterosexual epidemic could follow the outbreak among addicts, much as it did in Thailand, and devastate the population. The Health Ministry is determined to prevent this, and is actively studying the Thai response. The Thai program's successes have been due, in part, to the fact that Thai sexual behavior *had* been studied before the epidemic. Vietnam is just starting this process. The first major survey, done in collaboration with CARE International, confirmed some of these anxieties. Vietnamese men, northern and southern, *do* patronize sex workers, especially before marriage, on a fairly frequent basis: about one-third of all young men interviewed had paid for sex in the last year, and perhaps one-fifth of married men had done so. In another CARE-supported study of urban men, 54% of 1,100 interviewed reported sex with two or more partners in the previous two weeks. That is a lot of sex. Sex with other men was also reported fairly commonly; about 7% of men reported having had sex with another man; most of these men were married. But what was more disturbing was the lack of communication these men reported with their wives and girlfriends. Almost none had discussed extra-marital sex with their wives. Extensive focus-group discussions with married women, also done by CARE, found a commonly shared sense of powerlessness, an inability to confront husbands about their behavior. Fear of violence, of desertion, and of HIV, was widespread, a situation strikingly like that of women in Thailand, many of whom also live in fear of contracting HIV from their husbands and also feel incapable of discussing these fears with their men.

Whatever else can be said about highly centralized governments, they can mount impressive national campaigns. If Cambodia represents the difficulties of HIV prevention in a chaotic social order, Vietnam is an example of how a pervasive state can reach every corner of a diverse country and get a message out. HIV prevention is one message the Party has embraced. Vietnam is a country studded with AIDS information, at traffic circles, on billboards, in the papers. There is a 30-part soap opera under development which deals with a large multi-generational family, in which the husband has HIV. Hundreds of interviews with men and women were done in developing scripts. The show will take on issues like married partners talking about sex, parents and teenagers dealing with condom use, fathers and sons, mother and daughters. In Hanoi, I visited the National Offices of the campaign and saw their current output. The fliers and posters have come a long way from the early 'AIDS kills!' message of

just a few years ago. One showed a very loving and tender photo of
two men in bed, with an admonition for men to use condoms as a
way of showing love. Another was an explanation of what HIV
looks like in the early phases, with a photo of a late beloved friend,
the beautiful Tina Chow, in the asymptomatic stage of HIV. Tina
was one of the first Asian-American supermodels, and later a jewelry
designer. She is one of the most prominent American women to
have been felled by AIDS, and as fitting an image for the pathos and
beauty of lost lives as could be imagined. HIV education partly
follows the Thai model, going into schools, workplaces, and the mass
media. But whether relations with sex workers, with men in gay
bars, or with addicts, are as intimate and supportive is another matter.
This is not known. Given the party's legalism and puritanism, it is
unlikely. Official documents and educational materials still focus on
the 'control and eradication of social evils'.

Hanoi

Ho Chi Minh City, and to a lesser extent Hanoi, are already a bit
like Bangkok: big and bustling and growing at dizzying speed, too
fast, perhaps, for the liking of the party. Like China and Laos,
Vietnam's Communist Party is still very much the only political power
in the land. To be part of China's highest elite you have to have
been on the Long March. To be a part of Vietnam's, you have to
have cut your teeth fighting the French or the Americans. This means
that the men in question are no longer young; the three paramount
leaders are all over 75. The current balance of power is toward the
reformers in the party, but this could change. There is talk of
promoting younger men and women to positions of power. But the
Eighth Party Congress, in June 1996, opted for continuity rather
than change. The Politburo simply closed the country to tourists
during the Congress, as though their workings still required secrecy
in the age of CNN. That this would be a disaster for the thousands
of small business people who were reliant on the growing tourist
trade was not a consideration. Most of the tourist trade (and small
businesses) are in the south. The elderly men calling the shots are
not.

It is also true that the people organizing the national HIV data
are in Hanoi, not Saigon. When I showed a colleague (who knows

Vietnam well) the government's numbers, she immediately suggested that the drastic difference between the north and south could simply be due to differences in testing and reporting. It seems very unlikely that these data are 'cooked' in the sense of having been falsified or corrupted. But it is perhaps not unlikely that more extensive testing has been done in the south than in the north. The north is certainly not without risks. In Hanoi I never left my hotel without being offered a woman for the night by cyclo-drivers, cabbies, waiters, or barmen. I don't know if the locals can afford the sex, but for a Western man it is depressingly easy to find.

In Hanoi I spent some time with a doctor friend who had visited our project in Thailand. Dr B___ is a young and talented physician, his wife a nurse. Both are civil servants. Together they earn about US$70 a month, barely enough to eat. They are helped along by Dr B's mother, a retired teacher of English, who has a small state pension. Dr B, his wife, his mother, the couple's two children, and a nephew they are helping to raise live in one room in Hanoi. It is the front room of their family's old house. The family is passionate about education. Though his mother was a widow with very limited resources, she saw her son through medical training on her teacher's salary. Dr B could make more with a private clinic, but he is dedicated to research on Dengue fever, and this requires his staying at his Institute, which receives help from Sweden, and is arguably the best hospital for infectious diseases in the country. (The Swedes and the Finns were the only Western nations to support health care in North Vietnam during the war with the US.) Dr B remains grateful for their help. He would like to do advanced training himself, but is already saving for the education of his children and his nephew.

Dr B was a child during the bombing of Hanoi.

Yes, it was very frightening. We hid in the basement when the bombs came. We had to try to keep going to school. My mother kept trying to go to work. Once I was alone when a heavy raid came to this neighborhood. I will never forget it. Some of my schoolfriends died. But that is all in the past. We are free now and we have better relations with America, which we want. I don't like thinking about pains and fears from the past. They are behind us. Better that way! We have to go forward and develop our country.

What did Dr B think about the HIV problem in Vietnam?

We are going to need help. We are weak in epidemiology. My professor here is very good but he studied in Hungary, all of his books are in Hungarian. Difficult! We have to get more software, learn to analyze on computers. We have a long way to go. This HIV problem is very new to us; people are still very limited in their understanding. We know so little about what is happening in the countryside. I know we will see cases in children. We will. But we're not sure we will diagnose these correctly. And we are not sure we can afford to treat them. You have to understand how poor a country is Vietnam.

Societies in transition are, by definition, unbalanced. They can be both hopeful and threatening. Rapid growth is painful. Injustices resolve, if they do, unevenly. Thailand has made strides in freedom of thought and speech, but its legal system lags dangerously, and its police are unreformed and corrupt. Vietnam is not hungry, there are more 'things', but the life of the mind and the life of the spirit remained fettered. The Communist Party has the infrastructure, and the people, to mount impressive education and health programs, and it has done so. But the spiritual void that drives men and women to liquid opium, to buy and sell their precious physical selves, is less addressed. And this void will not be easily filled by education campaigns. Or, to use an adage, not by bread alone. Still, Vietnam is acting on AIDS, using the Thai example as a model. It may be able to prevent a disaster.

8. Yunnan: China's Southeast Asia

Prostitution and whoredom is an evil social phenomenon which was wiped out in the continent of China. Since 1980, however, not only the phenomenon was reappeared, but also there has been a rapid increasing imputors. According to statistics of the prostitutes and their clients from 1982 to July 1994, the accumulating number was 1.3 million. But, as estimated by the Department of Public Security, it was only part of the actual picture. HIV, which will be developed into AIDS at the later stage and is one of the sexually transmitted diseases like syphiliis and gonorrhea, has spread along with prostitution practice in the country and the development is with a rather rapid speed.

Ministy of Health, People's Republic of China

The Province of Yunnan is the cradle of the T'ai language family. The modern Thais, Laos, the Shans of Burma, the Assammese, and the ethnic Dai who still live in Yunnan are all branches of this T'ai linguistic tree. The region in southern Yunnan called Xishaung Banna by the Chinese, and Sip Song Pan Na by Thai speakers, is held to be the birthplace of the T'ai. 'Sip Song Pan' means twelve thousand, 'Na' means fields, so this is the land of twelve thousand (rice) fields. (Lan Na, the old name for northern Thailand, is the 'million rice fields'.) Northern Thais, but not central Thais, can still be understood in this part of Yunnan if they use their old dialect. This linguistic connection, and the cultural and historical links which years of political isolation have not destroyed, are taking on new importance as Yunnan is increasingly drawn into the development plans of the Southeast Asian community.

What unites Yunnan, Tibet, Burma, Laos, Thailand, Cambodia, and Vietnam is the great Mekong River. In Yunnan it is called the Lancang, an echo of the Kingdom of Lan Xang (million elephants), which once controlled much of what is now southern Yunnan and Laos. The Silk Road followed the Mekong through Yunnan, the Shan states, and across Laos to Huay Sai where it delved into

Thailand. This route once brought traders from across Asia into
Thailand. Chinese laborers now use the Mekong to get to Laos to
find work. This old leg of the silk route now carries perhaps 40% of
the world's heroin from Burma and Laos into Yunnan. The route
links the Burma road with the China road, crossing the Mekong on
the Burma–China border near Kachin state. It is along this route
that 80% of HIV infections in China have been found, and 60% of
all China's reported AIDS cases. Most of the infections have been
among young rural men; heroin addicts of the Kachin, Wa, and Dai
(T'ai) ethnic minorities. Further south, in Sip Song Pan Na, the HIV
cases are in ethnic Dai girls who have returned from sex work in
Thailand. The fact that these girls speak a dialect close to northern
Thai, coupled with their poverty and lack of education, has made
this part of Yunnan a trafficking center for the sex industry. Taken
together, these links suggest that the one major HIV outbreak seen
so far in China is very much a part of the wider Southeast Asian
epidemic. Yunnan, because of its history, location, and its ethnic
peoples, is showing its true face to China in the mirror of AIDS; it is
not a Han face.

Once a road, a river route, or a border opens, all manner of
things begin to flow. In this region, guns, girls, antiques, heroin, rice,
labor, jade, timber, rhino horns, tiger parts, tribal people in search
of land: the list is a long one. Two years ago virtually all the antiques
in the markets of Chiang Mai were Shan. Whole Shan temples,
dismembered and split into lots, were turning up in dealers' shops.
At the same time, nurses in clinics in northern Thailand were reporting that many of the new sex workers turning up with STDs were
Shan women and girls, mostly from around Keng Tung. The border
was unofficially open, and the road from Keng Tung to Tachilek to
Mae Sai on the Thai side was newly passable. The beautiful Shan
Buddhas were coming in the same trucks as the women.

In the dry season of 1994, curious wooden Buddhas with elongated
ears, arched eyebrows, and serene smiles began to appear. These
were folk carvings, not the highly finished Shan bronzes. While the
carving work was often delicately done, the proportions of the figures
were eccentric: heads too large, the hands and feet clumsy imitations
of Thai–Lao classical styles. Some were absolutely lovely, the folk
elements adding both charm and spirituality. Where were they from?
'Thai Lue' was the answer from the dealers, from the Dai ethnic

villages in Yunnan. Within a month of the appearance of the folk Buddhas, the nurses were again calling to say that a new group of girls and women were appearing in the clinics. Where were they from? Thai Lue, from Yunnan. Another route had opened, and a new trade in treasures, alive and not, was under way.

Not surprisingly, the countries of the Mekong region now call the river and its surrounding countryside a development zone. The plans include linking (with roads) northern Thailand, the Shan States of Burma, western Laos, and Yunnan, into a 'golden quadrangle' development area. The Asian Development Bank is supporting the idea, and the ASEAN states have done so as well. Perhaps development of this region will mean that legal goods and tourists, rather than heroin and young girls without passports, will travel the roads of the quadrangle. But the linkages may just as well mean that the last tigers, the last Buddhas in their village shrines, the last villages unreached by traffickers, will lose the protection of isolation and join the great regional boom, never to return.

China proper, by which I mean the Han lands and not the colonial holdings of the Party, also has an HIV problem, but the extent of HIV spread in the middle kingdom is currently a guessing game. At the 1995 China International Symposium on AIDS, held in Beijing in a bitter December, the numbers flew about like snow flurries, impossible to grasp. The official figure of reported cases was about 1,700, which everyone agreed was a gross underestimate. The WHO estimate was 10,000, based on a very low rate in what is a gigantic population. This figure was the result of work done by Dr James Chin, a respected researcher who was one of the participants. The Chinese Ministry of Health estimate was 100,000 HIV infections in 1995, based on little evidence, educated guesswork, and the bureaucrat's love of a round figure. A thousand? Ten thousand? A hundred thousand? After much discussion, a Party elder weighed in. The official estimate was to be 100,000 cases by 1995. Fact by decree.

When dealing with HIV in a population the size of China's, it may not matter how many cases you think there already might be – what can matter much more is how common the risk behaviors for HIV infection are among young adults. Is there much prostitution? How much injecting drug use is there outside Yunnan? How many gay and bisexual men are there? What is condom use like? How safe are medical procedures, the blood supply, dental care? But none of these questions is any more answerable than the estimates. And some, like the extent of prostitution or male–male sex, are questions with enormous political weight in China. If there are answers, who will be allowed to know them?

China has a very long history of sale and trade in women. In addition to outright sex workers there were always grey zones where sex and financial support were linked: minor wives, concubines, servants, the debt-bonded, slaves – all could be seen as part of a profoundly patriarchal system of the use of women for men's pleasure. To their credit, the communists saw this system as feudal and exploitative. One of their first social programs after consolidating power in 1949 was to 'eradicate' prostitution. Some four million women were 'rehabilitated' after deliverance from feudal orders. There is some evidence that this extreme program came close to eliminating STDs in China. Certainly prostitution, to whatever extent it continued to exist, became relatively rare when compared to the Warlord or Nationalist periods.

All of this is changing in the economic explosion of China in the 1990s. Everyone needs money, wants money, wants it now. Women with beauty are selling it again. Hotel lobbies are full of hostesses; bars and nightclubs have leggy women in short dresses working the crowd; Karaoke waitresses are 'available', and Karaokes are everywhere. Traffickers are back and are milking the rural poor for their daughters. Cross-border trade in women and girls is a reality. At the symposium, scattered bits of data suggested that syphilis, gonorrhea, herpes, and several other diseases spread through sex were coming back as well. This phenomenon is quite predictable, and likely to increase, despite the resistance of the party to sexual behavior outside monogamous marriage. The one-child policy has skewed China's population strongly in favor of males; the youngest age groups are now at something like 116 boys to every 100 girls, and thus the demand for women exceeds the supply. Men will be increasingly willing to pay for sex, as the odds on their finding a wife decline. Just as important is the need to appear rich and successful, which means providing hostesses for business dinners, and appearing at banquets with a beautiful girl or two on your arm.

Beijing is the showpiece of the China that now has as its chief slogan Deng Xiao-Peng's famous 'It is glorious to be rich'. The scale of the new city, imperviously trampling the old one, is monumental.

Virtually every corner sports a new hotel, shopping mall, or glistening bank.

At the symposium I met Dr Rosalyn Fon, an Australian whose family is from Hong Kong. Rosalyn runs AIDS Action in Hong Kong, which works with sex workers. She is a medical doctor with training in sexology, and had come to Beijing to find out the scope of the burgeoning commercial sex scene in the People's Republic. If you dreamed of a Chinese lady sexologist, you could not come up with Dr Fon. She is tall (5 feet 11 inches), curvaceous, with a highly set bust framed by Garbo shoulders and long white arms. Complete the vision with a serious pair of legs in black leather, stiletto pumps, a poly fur bomber, a shock of rag-doll red hair, dripping earrings and fire-engine lips and you have Rosalyn. The old PRC cadres literally gasped when she first appeared in a skin-tight mini-skirt at the opening ceremony in the Great Hall of the People.

After the first day's session, we agreed to go out on the town. The *Spartacus Gay Guide* had one listing for Beijing: a disco in the basement of yet another vast hotel. I did my best to dress for the occasion, and strode out of the awful 21st Century Hotel with the glamorous Dr Fon on my arm.

We arrived just before nine, and the place hadn't even opened. The disco shared the basement with a huge bowling alley. Dressed for night-clubbing, we watched bowling, a hypnotically dull game, and talked about Hong Kong. Would she stay after 1997?

'Well, I have an Australian passport, so I can get out if it looks bad. But I'm curious, you know, to see what it'll be like. Most Hong Kong people with money are investing in mainland China. They're really more concerned with their business ventures than with things like a free press and the vote. People are looking forward to not paying taxes to the Brits, I can tell you that. But there is one big worry with the PRC in charge, and that's corruption. Hong Kong isn't perfect, but you really do have to be very clever to get ahead, and the best people *do* get ahead. In China it's still who you know, whose kid you are, and who you can pay off to get promoted. Hong Kong people are worried not so much about communism, which is pretty much dead anyway, but about having some party chief's idiot son in charge of their business.'

On to the Disco. Most of the crowd looked like other Westerners who had read *Spartacus*. There was one rather stunning male couple rocking out on the dance floor. They turned out to be well-heeled tourists from New Delhi (and very much in love). Rosalyn and I met one gay Chinese, actually from Beijing but living in Sydney. I mentioned the rather obvious number of attractive young women in revealing dresses scattered throughout the club.

'Yeah, they're working girls. If a club in Beijing doesn't have them, no customers will come. You find them everywhere.'

'Are they hostesses, or do they sell sex as well?'

'You want one, isn't that lady your wife?'

'No, she's not my wife, just a friend. I'm gay, actually. I'm just interested.

'Of course, they will go home with you. If they didn't, this place couldn't make any money. Beijing people are very cheap; they don't spend money on drinks like the Aussies.'

Rosalyn listened to all this with a slight, bored smile. She had spent several years trying to get the Hong Kong authorities to acknowledge the scale of sex services in Hong Kong and on the mainland, and this was old territory for her. In the cab going back, I asked her about the commercial sex scene. How extensive did she think it was?

'In China now, all the old status symbols are coming back. It's in the genes! The people here have been denied so much for so long. Now they want it all: cars, luxuries, clothes. Sex is just a part of the money-and-power game. And let's face it, things have never been that great for women in China, even at the height of the communist reforms. HIV is a time-bomb here. Talk to the women in the bars, the young executives, they'll all tell you that you get AIDS only from sleeping with foreigners.'

'What about Hong Kong?'

'Officially there are only a small number of cases. The government likes to think that prostitution is uncommon. I've interviewed so many sex workers, and so many of them have repeated bouts of STDs, it just doesn't jibe with the official reports. Hong Kong does have something of a gay scene, though. There are some clubs and discos. We'll just have to see how things are handled when the transfer happens.'

Try the toads

The Chinese AIDS symposium was fascinating, not least because it was sponsored by two very different organizations: the China Academy of Traditional Chinese Medicine, and the China AIDS Foundation. The first is China's national body for research into traditional medicine; the second is Western (allopathic). The government made it clear at the symposium that China could not afford Western anti-viral therapies for people with AIDS (AZT, ddi, ddc, the protease inhibitors). Instead, China would focus on research using its traditional herbal (and animal and mineral) pharmacopeia. These treatments were also being used by some people with AIDS in the West: New-Agers, but also PWAs who either found western treatments intolerable, or found the Chinese concepts of harmony and balance in healing more compelling than biomedical approaches.

The China Academy has already had considerable experience in treating people with HIV/AIDS using their traditional therapies, although not in China. Since 1987 they have collaborated with the government of Tanzania in a large treatment scheme; they report having treated more than 10,000 Tanzanians with HIV, and claim considerable success, although their results are unpublished, at least in Western medical literature. It would certainly be of great interest to know how traditional therapies fared in Africa, where their herbal components might actually be affordable, in contrast to Western ones. This is made difficult, however, by the challenge of using scientific methods to evaluate traditional treatments, and by problems with research methodologies.

The research methods used by the traditionalists are an interesting mix of East and West. From a purely scientific-methods perspective, they are generally very weak: mixed methodologies that are neither fish nor fowl. One example might suffice. A senior researcher from the Academy of Traditional Medicine reported his investigations into the use of a traditional remedy as an anti-retroviral agent. He used as a model SIV, the simian immunodeficiency virus, a cousin of HIV that causes a fatal immune destruction, SAIDS, in some monkey species. SAIDS has many features in common with human AIDS, though not all. The researcher injected over 100 macaque monkeys with SIV, then fed half of them a traditional Chinese medicine composed of several plants. The other half of the sample were not given the medicine, and served as controls. He waited six weeks, sacrificed all the monkeys in both groups, harvested their lymph nodes, and used pathologic slides of these tissues to compare treated and untreated animals. It was a large experiment and an interesting idea. But the results were impossible to evaluate or understand.

SIV usually kills monkeys much more quickly than HIV kills most humans, but it is still a 'lentivirus', a slow virus, as HIV is. Monkey researchers must wait 6–12 months after introduction of SIV to understand what is happening. By sacrificing all the animals in what was actually the acute phase of infection, the most important data were immediately lost. Lymph-node biopsies have proved extremely valuable in understanding the early phase of HIV infection, so the choice of lymph-node tissues was a good one in this study. However, gross pathology, especially in the very short term, is a hopeless way to investigate efficacy. We all sat staring at hundreds of purplish blobs, one monkey node after another, and no one could interpret their meaning. It became a ghoulish Rorschach game, and was a sad waste of the monkeys' lives – the control monkeys in particular – and the researcher's efforts. Five would have been sufficient to show that the virus used in the challenge was indeed viable and could cause disease. This is another example of 'pseudo-science': the researcher simply borrowed the clinical trial method of an equal number of cases and controls for what was not, owing to its very short duration, a clinical trial. And then there is the problem of the treatment. How do you get monkeys to eat traditional medicine? Did they all eat it, or only some? And how much? To make any comparison, even on the weak lymph-node test, this would have been essential information.

There are other examples, but my personal favorite was a paper combining several classical techniques with a touch of Western science and a touch of shamanism. One group had investigated the acupuncture points associated with stimulation of the immune system. Arguing that as HIV was a disease of immune suppression (there are some who would argue that it is not, but rather a disease of immune activation gone awry), they sought a more potent method for activating these key points. It turns out that there is a toad in China that secretes potent toxins through its skin. This is not unusual for amphibians; many use toxins, potent nauseants, or other compounds as biologic weapons to dissuade predators. Some species produce compounds that are psychoactive in human brains as well; touching these live toads is used by some South American native shamans in trance induction. The Chinese solution was to use white linen cords to bind live toads to the acupuncture points thought to stimulate immunity. This team had some extraordinary photos of smiling AIDS patients wrapped in croaking bandages. I was sitting in the audience, incredulous, when a Thai colleague leaned over and said, 'You know, we have a lot of those toads in Chiang Mai.' So perhaps this therapy will spread.

The Western-tradition scientists from China are another matter. I met several people who were formidably bright and doing important work in virology, epidemiology, and vaccine research. One was clearly a genius. Dr Ximing Shao had been recommended by a Chinese-American colleague at Johns Hopkins as the key person to meet in Beijing. He was one of the first members of the WHO's technical advisory group on HIV vaccines, and has since developed a collaboration with a German group to develop HIV vaccines in China. After a quick lunch on the second day of the meeting with Dr Ximing, I felt, for the first time in ages, renewed optimism for the vaccine effort. The clarity of his ideas was wonderfully refreshing. He was convinced that a vaccine including core and envelope gene products could protect against HIV. He detailed his study plan; it was cohesive and logical, but also visionary. In the new China, he has official sanction for his work.

The last day of the meeting included a surprise guest. We assembled to meet the former head of the PRC Ministry of Health, a very senior Communist official. He had arrived to sign a new research agreement with a French counterpart. This was Dr Luc Montagnier, the *Institut Pasteur* researcher in whose lab HIV had first been isolated. There was considerable excitement among the Chinese participants as Montagnier announced the new initiative: his Institute and the Chinese Academy of Traditional Medicine were going to collaborate on investigating Chinese medical treatments for HIV infection and AIDS. This may be a fruitful marriage, perhaps a politically expedient one, but there is no doubt that China's ancient pharmacopeia deserves quality scientific investigation.

My translator at the seminar spoke on the second day. He was Dr Zunyou Wu, a young medical doctor with a Ph.D from UCLA, and a key member of the team investigating the epidemic of HIV among the Kachin (*Jingpo* in Mandarin) and Wa of Yunnan. He had some extraordinary slides of Kachin heroin users injecting each other with pens, bamboo splits, and razor blades. He later showed me a map of the epidemic in Yunnan. The cases were clustered in just three small districts, all along the China–Burma border. Sixty percent of all the infections in this immense country were in this one tiny area. He also had some slides of the Wa communities. If anything, these people were living in an even earlier epoch than the Wa in Burma, who had been penetrated by Burmese Communists in the 1960s. The Wa in Yunnan were still in loincloths, still hunting and fishing in their remote mountains, terribly vulnerable, as tribal peoples often are, to exploitation and drugs. Among the Kachins in Ruili, the border district in Yunnan, 17% of young men on either side are drug users, according to Dr Zunyou.

Information on the mandatory 're-education' programs used by the Yunnanese authorities to treat ethnic addicts is not available. It seems, however, not to be working. Certainly the HIV data shows an epidemic in poor control, and there are already a number of pregnant women – wives of addicts – infected. Still, it is nowhere near as grave a situation as in Kachin state on the Burmese side, where 91% of addicts tested HIV-positive in 1995, and where the virus has already leapt out of the addict circle and into the general population. This is not what the beleaguered Kachins need as they struggle with the SLORC.

Is what is happening among the ethnic minorities in Yunnan going to affect the Middle Kingdom? China is still not a very mobile society: people wait years for apartments; lovers postpone marriage for years until they can manage to get jobs in the same city. Social and sexual mixing of the Han and the ethnic populations is still uncommon. Tribal Wa, only a generation away from their last headhunts, are probably not going to work as Karaoke hostesses in Shanghai, at least not in any significant numbers. The greater threat to China is its own resurgent sex industry, its new consumer society, and its rapidly widening disparities in income, which will make selling sex attractive to the poor. With China's strict family-planning laws and extensive network of contraceptive services, it is somewhat ahead of the game. But the future is not at all certain.

Part Two
People, Risks

9. Women: wives, mothers, daughters

The basic strategy for the prevention of sexual transmission of HIV has comprised three messages: reduce the number of your sex partners (toward monogamy, if possible); use condoms every time you have penetrative intercourse; promptly treat all sexually transmitted diseases (STDs) and reduce (with condoms and partner reduction) your risk of acquiring new STDs. This strategy grew out of prevention efforts by and for gay men, with the 'sex negative' input of bodies like the US Centers for Disease Control (CDC), which was mandated to include promotion of monogamy in its messages. And it has worked, albeit with varying degrees of success. This triple approach has also had some utility for sexually active heterosexual adults and adolescents, largely in the West, and for sex workers and their clients in many countries. For people with multiple sex partners by choice, HIV risks can be sharply reduced by adhering to consistent condom use and STD treatment.

Now imagine yourself a young married woman, in Thailand or Cambodia, Burma or Malaysia. You have only one sex partner, your husband. He is your sexual life. Your risks are his risks. You may or may not know what they are. You may or may not be able to ask. 'Reducing the number of sex partners' means not having sex with him, and thus, not at all. This is not an option for many women, no matter what their husband's behavior entails. It would mean giving up having children, an option very few women can accept, particularly among the rural poor, still the vast majority of Asians, for whom the focus of life itself is the family. 'Use condoms for penetrative sex.' Why? Why introduce condoms into your marriage? Condoms again represent your husband's risks, and again imply reduced fertility. Using them acknowledges that he *has* risks, has other partners, goes to brothels or has a mistress or sleeps with men or

injects drugs. And *he* has to put the condom on, has to accept the
need to protect you from his behavior. (Thai men, for example,
usually report using condoms with sex workers to protect themselves,
recognizing their own risk. The acknowledgement that as a user of
commercial sex services they could spread HIV to others is unusual.)
'Reduce the risk of STDs' is another ambiguous message for most
women. If they get gonorrhea, or syphilis, it is, again, their husband's
behavior that is at issue. What can a woman do about reducing her
partner's risks for STDs, or his need for treatment? To speak of
these issues is to suggest infidelity. This can be frightening. It can be
deadly.

If this scenario seems an unlikely or uncommon one, it may be
because we're used to thinking of HIV in terms of 'high-risk sex'.
Anal intercourse aside, there is no higher-risk sexual activity for HIV
than trying to conceive a child. It requires regular unprotected
intercourse, the exchange of just those fluids that carry and transmit
HIV. Death and life in one ejaculate, a parasitic mechanism of
'fearful symmetry'. Wives outnumber sex workers by many orders of
magnitude in all of the countries in this study. Probably in every
society. By far the most common risk factor for HIV among women
in Thailand is marriage, the having of one male partner. This is
already true in India, in Burma, and in much of Africa. How else
can we explain the report of the Myanmar National AIDS Program
that 175,000 pregnant women in Burma were already HIV-infected
by 1995? These are not addicts, or 'loose women', or sex workers,
though a small minority may be. These are women whose HIV
exposure comes from just the behaviors their society most strongly
supports: marriage, conception, giving birth to children.

We have very little to offer women in this situation, the bulk of
people now most at risk worldwide. The male condom is problematic.
It is strongly associated with prostitutes, 'risky' sex and 'risky' partners, mistrust, and sex without love or commitment. A married
woman in Malaysia or Thailand would probably be mortified to buy
one. The female condom may be an improvement, but it is expensive,
still requires male consent for use, shows outside the vulva, and
requires that a woman be willing to insert it. Many Asian women are
psychologically unable to touch themselves internally. Many have
never had a gynecological examination. *Our Bodies, Ourselves* has not
been translated into Shan, or Lao, or Punjabi.

Looking at another gynecological disease may help to illustrate these challenges. Cervical cancer in women is a growing problem worldwide. It has been linked to another sexually transmitted agent, HPV, the human papilloma virus, which can cause genital warts in men and women. Women with only one lifetime sex partner are exposed to HPV by that partner. But HPV is tricky, like HIV. HPV-infected men often have no symptoms, although when they do, the warty lesions of penile HPV are unmistakable. In Thai they are called 'Nok Kai' the cock's comb, which they do somewhat resemble, and are one of the few STDs with such a precise folk translation. Cervical cancer is unusual among gynecologic cancers in that we have a cheap and effective screening test, the Pap smear, for early detection. Caught in the first stages, this is a curable disease. Despite the relative ease and low cost of Pap smears, they are rarely done in developing countries. Most cervical cancer in Thailand, the only Southeast Asian country for which we have reasonable data, is found in later, less treatable stages, or at incurable ones. Pap smears are not done routinely because pelvic examinations are not done routinely. Sex workers get pelvic examinations to look for STDs. Housewives and mothers do not. It should not come as a surprise to find that cervical cancer is the leading cause of cancer death among Thai women -- all women, not just sex workers.

When we think of protecting women from HIV, now an incurable infection, this reality has to be kept in mind. Limitations on women's health care in much of Asia have already led to a serious failure of prevention for a common and potentially curable disease. HIV will be no easier to prevent than cervical cancer. And, while both diseases are sufficient to kill a woman, their interaction is even more deadly. HIV-infected women progress to cervical cancer more quickly than women without HIV, and HIV-positive women are more likely to infect their sex partners with HPV, since the wart virus can grow without the hindrances of a healthy immune system. The viruses accelerate each other, a phenomenon Dr Judy Wasserheit of the CDC has called 'epidemiologic synergy'. (This synergy has also led to an increase in the number of cases of a previously rare disease, carcinoma of the anus, among men infected with both HIV and anal HPV.)

HIV exposes women's vulnerability to male sexual behavior. What can women do about it? How will women in Southeast Asia respond?

About 60 women meet each week at a Buddhist temple in Doi Saket district, Chiang Mai Province. Doi Saket was once a rural area, with a small country town and a number of farming villages. Urban sprawl has brought Doi Saket's farmers into the growing suburban economy; land has been sold for sub-divisions; many villagers commute to work in the city; young people leave Doi Saket early, for schooling and for work. These changes have brought some prosperity, but not without costs. The cash economy, and men and women leaving villages for work, have loosened social structures, separated families, changed women's lives. This period of social change, unfortunately, made Doi Saket, and other communities like it, fertile ground for HIV. All of the women who meet at the temple are AIDS widows. Many are themselves infected; most are now single mothers. Despite the fact that nearly all of the women in the widows' group were farmers' wives infected by their husbands, community prejudice and discrimination against them and their children has been intense. It was this social ostracism that first brought the group together. They approached the government, who helped them to get support from an Australian donor agency. With the money, the widows of Doi Saket have set up a co-operative, making handicrafts to support themselves and their children. The Abbot of the district's central *wat*, who has taken a lead in supporting people with HIV infection, offered the temple grounds for their projects. This is not an HIV prevention program, it is perhaps too late for early interventions here, but it is a way for women to survive the loss of their husbands, to deal with discrimination, and to build solidarity with each other.

The women of a similar community, also in the suburban ring of Chiang Mai, San Sai District, have used another approach. So many young men were dying in San Sai that the community opted for a moratorium on marriage until it was clear which young men would survive the disastrous HIV epidemic in the district. (Between one in five and one in four young men have died, or will die, if spread stopped tomorrow.) This is probably not going to work, but it represents an incredible change in the social structure of San Sai's villages. Local women know what may happen when they marry – HIV infection – and are opting, at least for the short term, for not marrying rather than risk exposure.

Women's attitudes toward prospective partners are changing as well. In a study among female factory workers in northern Thailand, young women reported that they strongly favored men who did not visit sex workers, and that the sexual history of their potential partners was an important criterion for marriage. This is a sharp change from the attitudes of their mothers' generation, for whom visits to sex workers were often preferred over husbands having mistresses. These were women whose fathers and older brothers traditionally took their adolescent boys to brothels to begin their sexual lives.

The most far-reaching change is a paradoxical one. Young Thai women are increasingly having sex before marriage. The formal term for this emerging pattern is 'serial monogamy'. In serial monogamy, people tend to have only one partner at a time, a steady monogamous partner. But the first, or second, or third partner might not be the one chosen for marriage. Serial monogamy is trial and error, learning, while engaged in sexual relationships, what one wants and is prepared to give to a marriage. This requires contraception, and an awareness on the part of both partners that neither is likely to be a virgin at marriage. It requires empowerment of young women and a sea-change for men, who must go from a 'virgin or whore' conception of female sexuality to a partnership with an 'equally experienced and adult' woman.

A striking finding among Thai soldiers was that while condom use was increasing sharply in the early 1990s, and the use of prostitutes steadily declining, the age at first intercourse among these men fell through the same period (from about 16.5 years to 16.1), and the number of men who reported having girlfriends with whom they were sexually active rose. The number of men who reported having had a girlfriend as their first sex partner (not a sex worker) more than doubled between 1991 and 1995. In other words, young Thai men were still having sex, but they were losing virginity and having sexual relationships with female peers, not sex workers. Does this mean that these 'AIDS era' young men may establish sexually satisfying lives with their wives? That prostitution will decline due to a fall in demand?

Many Islamic societies believe that sexual desire is a female problem. Women's genitals must be mutilated to prevent them from developing insatiable and uncontrollable craving. Men are seen as much less physical, more spiritual; if men were not constantly aroused

by licentious women they would spend their waking hours con-
templating the divine. *The Perfumed Garden,* the classical Arabic erotic
text, is a paean to women's 'itchy vulvas', their libidinous urges, and
the great lengths to which men must go in order to restrain their
women. Other cultures have seen this very differently. In Thai culture
wives traditionally do not enjoy or initiate sex, and do not have
orgasms. Sex workers are for sexual pleasure, wives for producing
heirs. A Western colleague and social researcher has done some
fascinating work on young women working in factories (women make
up about 70% of Thailand's factory workers). But it was with her
Thai research colleagues that she became intimate enough to en-
counter the sexual conservatism of middle- and upper-class married
Thai women of a certain age. She had her research group to her
house for tea near the completion of their project. The subject of
sex within their marriages came up. Every one of these women was
shocked when my friend mentioned that she and her husband had a
satisfying sexual relationship. What did she mean? That her husband
was satisfied? No, she explained, she meant that she was satisfied;
her husband was a generous partner. She had orgasms. *Orgasms*?!
Impossible. Women couldn't have orgasms. How could they ejaculate?
The Westerner insisted that women did have orgasms, and there was
considerable scientific evidence to prove it. (The Thais present were
all educators, physicians, or pharmacists.) When she maintained that
she enjoyed sex, the consensus was that there was something very
wrong with her. One colleague suggested therapy, while another
thought she should take up meditation, to calm her over-aroused
senses.

But the daughters of these women might tell you a very different
story, one that has been profoundly affected by AIDS. Sexual equality
(serial monogamy for both partners until a good match is found)
may seem an unlikely outcome of the HIV epidemic in Thailand,
but it is increasingly being practiced by young women who want to
be a part of their husbands' erotic lives, not just dutiful and sexless
mothers of children, who want to know their husbands' and their
own risks, and want protection. And their husbands come from a
new generation of young men, who have had their sexual debut with
a girlfriend, not in a brothel.

This may sound like a change for the better. And perhaps it will
be, in the long term, a partial solution to the related problems of the

sex trade and sexually unfulfilling marriages. But it is having another consequence. The large pool of young men infected with HIV during the Thai boom (a similar situation prevails in Burma and Cambodia, where the booms continue) is now marrying. Young women in these countries are selecting partners with at least a 10% chance of having HIV. In the upper classes of these societies, the odds will be much lower. For women from San Sai, or Doi Saket, or Phnom Penh or the Shan States, they will be higher. Antenatal care clinics, where women go for pregnancy testing and care, have become HIV-testing sites throughout the region. Malaysia carried out a study in pregnant women in the early 1990s, but the results have been deemed too sensitive to release. The HIV rate among pregnant women in Keng Tung, one of the larger Shan State towns, was over 10% in 1995. In Payao province, northern Thailand, it is over 18% – roughly one in five babies in this farming community is being born to a mother with HIV infection. AZT, which has recently been shown to be remarkably effective in preventing HIV transmission from mother to infant, is unavailable in Laos, Burma, Cambodia, much of Thailand, Vietnam, and Yunnan. It is available in Malaysia, though how much it is used is unknown.

The study that showed the efficacy of AZT (zidovudine) in pregnancy was called ACTG 076. In the study, HIV-infected women were randomized to two groups: half the women received AZT and half placebo. The regimen was a complex one: oral AZT for the mother in the last three months of pregnancy, intravenous AZT during labor, oral AZT for the infant for six weeks after birth. In women who did not get AZT the HIV infection rate among their babies was a predictable 25%. Among the treated mothers and babies, it was 7%, a striking and statistically significant difference. *It worked.* This study was funded by US taxpayers, through the National Institutes of Health. AZT remains an expensive drug, despite the fact that its manufacturer, the British company Burroughs Wellcome, has already made profits from its sales of the order of US$275 million per year in the early 1990s, when it was one of the few licensed agents.[1] It remains so expensive as to be unavailable to the people who now need it most – pregnant women in the developing world, who give birth to 95% of the babies at risk of HIV infection. (Average developing-country expenditures on health are about US$2 per person per year, the retail cost of about two AZT tablets in the

US.) If you looked for a clearer case in which First World economic considerations cause suffering in Third World settings you could find no more pernicious example than the exorbitant cost of AZT. If you have ever cared for a baby born with HIV infection, and watched its short, painful life ebb away, you know that there is no language too strong to describe this injustice. We know we can save hundreds of thousands of babies from this fate, but we cannot make the pharmaceutical industry yield on costs. If they don't yield, perhaps Asia's entrepreneurs, who have managed to copy so many other items the West has to offer, will copy AZT as well. If fifty-cent Madonna CDs can get to Vientiane, and ten-dollar Rolex watches sell in Chiang Mai, why not 'bootleg' AZT?

There are other, less radical, solutions as well. The regimen of 076, AZT in three formulations, might be simplified, and costs reduced. Studies jointly funded by the US and Thai governments are under way to look at alternative regimens for AZT in pregnancy. Perhaps the doses for new-born babies are unnecessary, or the intravenous infusion during labor not needed; if we could get the beneficial effect of AZT with a minimal dose at the right time, the drug might be affordable in some countries where it is unavailable now. But for the others? AIDS care in Burma is extra rice, Tylenol, and prayer. If AZT were free it would remain almost impossible to deliver, given the current state of health care under SLORC.

For AZT to be effective in pregnancy on a population level, HIV testing would have to be made widely available, and offered to all women at risk. If discrimination is not addressed, the increased HIV testing necessary to prevent HIV in infants could have disastrous effects. A whole generation of children born HIV-negative but to infected mothers will grow up under a cloud. Who will educate and support them? How will the societies in which they live cope with their manifold needs? This is a question of immense importance for Thailand, Burma, and Cambodia, which will have large numbers of AIDS orphans for at least another generation. It is a reality which makes the problems of AIDS among gay men look easy.

There were three of us in the car: myself, my Thai partner S, and his older sister, Khun O, a teacher. S shares a house with his sister, her husband, and their two pre-teenage children. We were on our way to visit a Buddhist shrine in a limestone cave north of Chiang

Mai, a place of pilgrimage. S and Khun O are both devout Christians, members of the Church of Christ in Thailand. They were taking me to the cave, but for them both it was a place of historical, not religious, significance. The conversation was mostly about the US – Khun O had just returned from a school trip with her students. Then we started talking about my work, and about the HIV problem in Thailand. I went into a long monologue on the current challenge: how to protect married women, the difficulty of condom use in marriage, the relative ease of dealing with commercial sex compared to dealing with sex in the home. The car became uncomfortably silent. I sensed I had overstepped the bounds of propriety, and by going on about Thai men's sexual behavior in the abstract, had insulted my friends. It was a relief to get to the cave. Khun O didn't want to join us on the long steep climb into the shrine; S and I went on alone. In the cave, I apologized to S. He stopped me cold:

'No, Chris. My sister couldn't tell you what's happening to her. I was waiting for her to tell you, but she can't. My brother-in-law has taken a minor wife. She thinks he's also going with other women, but she's not sure. She wants him back. We are very against divorce, you know? But she's very afraid. She wants me to go with her to get tested. Maybe in Bangkok. I told her I think he needs to get tested. But how to say?'

Note

1. For a detailed history of this controversial drug and its costs, see Randy Shilts's brilliant polemic, *And the Band Played On*.

10. The flesh trade: prostitution and trafficking in ASEAN

Trafficking in women consists of the transport, sale and purchase of women for the purpose of prostitution and bonded labor within the country of origin and abroad. This includes a variety of forms and practices under which women live and work in extremely oppressive and/or slave-like conditions.

Cambodian Women's Development Association

A brothel in Cambodia may offer women and girls trafficked from Cambodia, Thailand, Vietnam, China, or the Philippines. Cambodian women have been trafficked to Singapore, Hong Kong, Malaysia, and Thailand. A brothel in Thailand may have women and girls trafficked from rural Thailand, from Burma, China (Yunnan), Laos and Cambodia. Japan receives most of its trafficked women and girls from Thailand and the Philippines; as many as 50,000 Thai women may work there. India traffics mainly rural and tribal women and girls, as well as large numbers of Nepalese. Malaysia's sex trade has Cambodian, Thai and Burmese women, and Indonesians, in addition to Malaysians. Thai women have been found in sexual slavery in California and in Sweden. Vietnamese women have been found trafficked at sea, traded from ship to ship by pirates, homeless and stateless.

This is an industry, and a profitable one, as the African slave trade was profitable in its day. But unlike the legal trafficking of humans in the 17th–19th centuries, this form of slavery is untaxed and untariffed. Though illegal, it is low risk compared to trafficking in drugs, tolerated with the right kind of bribes, and offers attractive perks – free access to the merchandise. Trafficking supplies a service – cheap sex – for which there are always buyers. Demand is high in ASEAN countries, and growing as the regions' bullish economies grow, as gaps between rich and poor widen, as family and community bonds are transformed by rapid economic and social change.

The sex trade is a relatively small component of the current trade in illegal labor in ASEAN. The Thai Ministry of the Interior estimates that there are at least 500,000 illegal workers in Thailand, 375,000 of whom are thought to be Burmese and 100,000 from Laos. NGOs active with illegal workers put the number at closer to 1 million, of whom 750,000 are thought to be Burmese. Sex workers account for only a minority of these persons, 5–10% at the most. The majority of trafficked laborers work in construction, on road crews, as agricultural migrants, fishermen, loggers, and domestic servants. The same is true for Malaysia, which estimates that there are over 1 million illegal workers in a workforce of only 8 million, and where, again, sex workers would be a tiny minority of these laborers. But trafficking for the commercial sex industry results in human rights abuses on a different scale from most other forms of labor, and it has a much higher mortality rate. Commercial sex is at the heart of Southeast Asia's AIDS catastrophe. And sexual slavery reveals the darkest sides of the countries involved: the status and treatment of women, the power of criminality, the depth and pervasiveness of corruption, what people will do for money.

The Cambodian Women's Development Association estimates that in 1990 there were perhaps 1,500 sex workers and 224 brothel managers in Phnom Penh. A year later, as the country began to open up to the world, and to development aid, there were 6,000 sex workers. After a few months of the United Nations (UNTAC) presence in Cambodia, there were 20,000. Getting this many women into the sex trade requires trafficking, it requires the use of force, and it requires networks to get women from villages to brothels. A United Nations High Commission for Refugees (UNHCR) spokesman put it this way: '. . . while UNTAC is not responsible for creating Cambodia's current prostitution and trafficking problems, UNTAC's presence facilitated the creation of the apparatus [of trafficking] and the machine has circulated.'

How does the apparatus work?

The trade typically begins in a poor, remote place: an ethnic minority village in Yunnan, an impoverished farming community in northern Thailand, an Akha tribal homestead, or a Shan village caught in the crossfire of the Burmese civil war. About 40% of the women in the debt-bonded sex trade in northern Thailand are Shan women and girls. This is one of the better understood trafficking systems, thanks largely to NGO workers in Chiang Mai, one of the destination points for trafficked Shans.

Although abduction happens, as does outright sale of daughters among the poorest of the poor, the trafficking road usually starts with a job offer. A girl is offered work as a waitress, or a maid. Her family usually gets some money. In Thai villages the rate is 5,000–10,000 Baht, in Shan villages somewhat less. This is the start of the debt, and of the bondage. The woman and her family may or may not have an idea what their daughter is headed for, and they may not have many choices.[1] In Burma, the army comes through minority areas frequently in search of porters for their campaigns; two porters for every soldier is standard. Forced porterage in the mountains of Burma is often a death-sentence, and the only way out is to pay. In cash. And so daughters are sent to Thailand in an attempt to protect sons. Among hilltribe peoples such as the Akha and the Hmong, drug debts among fathers have been found to be the commonest reason for the sale of daughters. The networks which supply the heroin know only too well which households are in need of money, and whose daughters are ripe for purchase.

There is a limited number of trafficking routes into Thailand and all require bribes along the way. These are added to the debt. On arrival, the trafficker hands the girl over to a brothel agent. The debt is transferred to the agent. Here she will typically be sold as a 'virgin', whatever her experience. If the trafficker did not violate her already, the agent will. New arrivals are big money; she may not know this, and she may be sold as a 'virgin' twenty or thirty times at the beginning. This is serial rape. The breaking-in process, in which a woman must learn how hopeless her situation is, how little she can do about it, and what sex is. If she refuses, she is raped or beaten, often both. Some escape. Most, in shock, learn the ways of dissociation and forgetting. Then she is trafficked to her destination, a brothel somewhere – it may be in Chiang Mai, or Bangkok, Ranong, Phuket, Hat Yai, or farther afield. Here the debt is doubled.

Most trafficked women and girls arrive at their first workplace owing 10,000–20,000 Baht to the brothel owner. Their wages are further deducted for room and board, for clothes and makeup, sometimes for condoms, always for drugs to treat STDs and for contraception. After these deductions, a debt-bonded worker usually earns 15 Baht (about 70 cents) for each client she serves. It is with this money that she has to pay off the debt. It can easily take a thousand or more sex acts to pay it off. Many women never make it. Some, particularly tribal women, are innumerate and so cannot keep track of their debts and wages. These girls can get hopelessly mired in debt.

When a woman does, finally, break even, the owner is supposed to start paying her. This is often the time the owner will call the police for a raid. It will cost 3,000 Baht in bribes to get a woman without papers out of jail. The brothel owner will pay this, and the woman will be back in his or her debt. If she refuses, she may be taken to the one of the International Detention Centers (IDCs) for illegal immigrants, and from there 're-patriated', usually to the Thai–Burmese border. At the border she will face several options: she can try and get back home, risking Burmese army patrols, arrest, and more rape; or she could talk to the brothel agents, who just happen to be waiting in their pickup trucks. For a fee, they will take her back to another brothel, and she will be in debt again.

Trafficking is slavery of a particularly precarious kind. Most workers trafficked across national boundaries are illegal aliens, and essentially have no rights. Women trafficked into sex work are also criminals in the eyes of the law: the work they do is illegal in itself. They are subject to prosecution in Thailand, Malaysia, Cambodia, Singapore, and China, whether they have been forced into prosutition or not. As many as 10,000 such women come to Thailand each year. And this has increased, not decreased, as education programs have reached the Thai villages that used to supply sex workers. These communities have stopped sending their daughters to the sex trade because HIV has begun to devastate their young people. This has forced traffickers to go farther afield, to find communities – and there are many – where HIV is still a distant rumor, and a few thousand Baht looks like a fortune.

Isn't this illegal? Burma is supposed to be a closed country, with strict limitations on nationals traveling abroad. The plain truth is that a village girl from a remote part of Burma or China does not get to a nightclub in Phnom Penh or Bangkok without the collusion of officials at numerous points in the trafficking process. There are border patrols on both sides, immigration police at check points, and local police on arrival. Khun Anand, former Prime Minister of Thailand, has pointed to the police and the legal system as the two sectors in Thai society most in need of reform. His observations could be generalized to several neighboring countries. In Cambodia and Burma too, law enforcement is heavily affected by corruption; almost no one expects fairness from the police or justice from the courts, certainly no one without money or influence. Some of the largest sex venues in all three countries are operated by individuals from law enforcement sectors. The police are a national embarrassment to progressive Thais, but remain a powerful, if shadowy, force in society.

Buyers

Trafficking is the supply side of the sex industry. What about demand? Who is interested in having sex with a slave? One argument might be that men simply want as much sex as they can get, the terms less important than the release, the sex partner less important than the man's sexual gratification. Brothel sex is not about conversation. If you adhere to biological determinism, several hundred million years of evolution are behind the male drive to spread his DNA as widely as possible. The raising of human infants and children, however, requires long-term emotional stability, the socio-biologists' 'pair bond'. Societies, as Freud argued, have to find ways of balancing the archaic, potent force of sexual desire with the maintenance of socially valued structures: marriage, the family, kinship ties, and now 'sexual health'.

Social solutions to this dilemma vary widely: Muslim Java allows young men the sexual outlet of transvestites; sexual experimentation with male peers is common in many cultures. The modern West, in some settings and social classes at least, tolerates young adult sex before marriage, for boys and, increasingly, for girls. In mainland Southeast Asia, by far the most common sexual outlet for men is the use of sex workers, trafficked or not. This was also the case in China before the communist revolution, and it is still true in India, though vigorously denied.

In the Thai case, widespread prostitution has allowed Thai men the valued sexual freedom they enjoy while protecting the majority of unmarried women from sexual experience. Structurally, prostitution creates a sub-class of women who fulfill the unmet sexual needs of men, while allowing the society to maintain equally valued female virginity, female monogamy in marriage, and clear lines of inheritance for family wealth. The children a man may father with a prostitute are her problem, not his. Prostitution also allows poorly educated women to fulfill their duties in supporting parents. In its modern form it allows low-income families to build the new cement houses that say so much to their communities about status, modernity, and class. It can be, for the minority of women who succeed at it, a lucrative form of employment. And it can be slavery.

The demand side of commercial sex in Asia is sharply delineated by class. The play of money and power in the sex trade isn't just between clients and workers, but between wealthy men and poor men. The rich can get fantasy: time with a beautiful and skilled creature who will do their bidding, and who may be making a reasonable living. In studies in Thailand the majority of higher-priced sex workers are divorced women, not trafficked, and often self-employed. Poor men get a raw reality: 30 minutes maximum (usually less) with a frightened trafficked girl on a damp bed. The cheapest sex in Chiang Mai is 40 Baht, less than a bottle of beer. Cambodia and Burma are cheaper still, a woman in upper Burma can be had for 5 Kyat, less than a nickel on the black market. Yet an hour with a Russian woman in Bangkok can cost 3,000 Baht, a 'virgin' up to 10,000. HIV also segregates along class divisions. At a 40-Baht brothel in northern Thailand, up to 70% of the women are HIV-infected. In the best massage parlors (some are owned by doctors), less than 2% may be positive. For wealthy clients condoms are a trivial expense. For the poorest men, they may substantially increase the cost of sex. This is why Thailand must be applauded for distributing 60 million free condoms per year, and helping to decrease at least the financial barriers to safer sex.

We know less about users of the sex trade in Burma, though commercial sex is generally thought to be less extensive than in Thailand, with the important exception of the gem mines of the Shan and Kachin states, where there are reported to be very large, if covert, numbers of brothels. HIV infection rates among Burma's sex workers in 1994 were high, at an average of perhaps 17% across the country, but widespread testing has not been done. It is a much more dangerous undertaking for a Burmese man to visit a sex worker than for a Thai man to do so. Burmese men who visit prostitutes can be charged under the British penal codes of 1886, which make the use of prostitutes equivalent to rape, and carry up to 10-year prison sentences. Careers and reputations can be ruined by such charges. These laws are reportedly rarely enforced, and never against SLORC or its people. But they can be used against enemies of the junta, another component of the mechanics of fear. The effect of these stiff penalties has been to drive commercial sex in Burma deep underground. A friend who recently conducted a health consultation in Burma, which included attempting to look at commercial sex, had this to say:

> There are few formal 'brothels' as such, because these are too easily detected. Instead, men typically contact pimps along certain roads, who then bring girls to their cars. Several men will usually share one woman for a night, with some finding the woman, and others a room to use, which is often more difficult. Each man in the group then has a 'turn' of sex with the sex worker. This informal and fluid system of commercial sex makes education and outreach to the women involved virtually impossible.

Sex is cheap in Burma, but social and health risks are high. Prostitution, like drug use, appears to have sharply increased under SLORC. A journalist who recently attempted to investigate this phenomenon talked to several sex workers in Rangoon, Mandalay, and Keng Tung. He met a 17-year-old Burmese girl whose mother had sold her to a brothel agent to feed the other children in the family. The girl charged 20 Kyat (about 15 cents) for sex, 100 Kyat for a full night. A full night's work means that the customer is allowed to bring his friends. She had just spent the night with a man and twelve of his friends, each of whom had had intercourse with her twice – 26 acts of penetration in a seven-hour period. For this, she earned less than a dollar.

Given the social 'benefits' of sex work, the release it allows men and the 'protection' prostitution affords the other women in a society, it is striking that so many of the societies that use this mechanism consider sex work so shameful, and that sex workers should be so marginalized. The Cambodians have an expression which captures this attitude: 'If the skirt is torn, do not tear it further', meaning that if a woman has been 'spoiled' she should keep it secret; it should never be made public. Prostitution is illegal in every country in

Southeast Asia, including Thailand. Most women involved in the ASEAN regional sex industry have virtually no rights as workers, and it is they, not owners or managers, who typically suffer harassment from the law. There has been only one successful prosecution of a brothel owner in the 36 years since prostitution became illegal in Thailand. This was the owner of a brothel in Phuket which suffered a disastrous fire, in the wreckage of which were found the bodies of two young girls who had been chained to their beds. The case took eight years to prosecute.

All of these difficulties seem small when HIV enters the picture. It becomes the ultimate occupational hazard. What do you think the odds are of avoiding HIV infection through hundreds or thousands of sex acts in countries where between one in ten and one in five men penetrating you will be carrying the virus? In India, in Thailand, in Cambodia, the women who serve the sexual needs of men are at extraordinary risk of HIV: more than half will get it in these countries. It needn't be so.

In the handful of countries where sex work is legitimate and sex workers have civil and worker's rights, they have impressively low HIV rates. Nevada, the one US state where prostitution is not a crime, has among the lowest HIV rates among sex workers in the US. Dutch sex workers are unionized, protected by the law, and empowered to refuse clients who want unsafe sex. HIV infection among these women is unusual. But legalizing (or decriminalizing) sex work means accepting that prostitution is part of your society, that men want it and will use it if available. Moralistic and legalistic approaches, while clear public health failures, have been by far the most common social response to prostitution. There are 49 US states with laws very different from Nevada's. Laws against sex work in Asia, like those in the US, have done virtually nothing to protect women, but have worked well to allow considerable profits for criminal trafficking operations, and have, the evidence suggests, facilitated the spread of HIV.

Natural immunity

One of the burning questions in current HIV research is natural immunity. There is some evidence that some individuals may be, due to genetic or other factors, resistant to infection with HIV. This has vital implications for vaccine research: if the body already has a way of preventing HIV infection, then we may have a model for designing a vaccine. The first two studies to report this possibility were from Africa, and they were both done in female sex workers. For the heterosexual epidemics of HIV in Africa and Asia, women in the sex trade have become what gay men with multiple partners have been for the homosexual epidemic, a key study population. They represent a core group with extraordinarily high risks for HIV and other sexual pathogens. Their large number of partners and sex acts means that preventive measures can be evaluated much more quickly than among women with only one partner, and fewer sex acts. The sexual acts that happen in brothels, with a woman having multiple different sex partners in a single night, may, however, be biologically very different from sex in the context of marriage. Vaginal flora change. Birth-control practices often differ. Other sexually transmitted diseases are many times more common in sex workers. A woman married to an HIV-infected man may be exposed to low levels of virus in his semen, if he is healthy and in the asymptomatic phase. Indeed many such women remain HIV-negative despite repeated exposure. Sex workers are exposed to men at all stages of HIV infection, including what may be the most infective period of all, the first few months after exposure. Taken together, these differences make sex work an uncertain model for heterosexual transmission of HIV. For studying possible resistance to the virus, however, these same biologic attributes make sex workers ideal.

Two studies of resistance to HIV in Africa have identified small groups of women who, by virtue of their many sex partners, low condom use, and multiple other sexually transmitted diseases, should have become HIV infected, but didn't. One group found six such women in Gambia; the other, 25 in Kenya. Our research group wanted to explore whether this phenomenon was also present in Thai women working in the sex trade. We studied women who also had many partners in a setting where one in ten of their customers may be HIV-positive. We searched our records and identified a handful of women who met these criteria. One was working in a brothel outside a small city, about 40 kilometers from Chiang Mai. The records showed that she had worked in brothels for 9 years, since 1986, before the epidemic started, and before condom use was common. We'll call her Khun Noi.

Khun Noi told us she had had, on average, 4 customers a day, more on festivals and paydays. She usually worked 20–25 days per month, which adds up to more than 10,000 sexual contacts after 9 years. She had had gonorrhea several times a year over this period, syphilis twice, had been treated for recurrent venereal herpes and had been pregnant twice, but had never become infected with HIV. The odds were wildly against this outcome, and a biologic basis for her lack of infection looked plausible.

I went with the nurses from the provincial STD clinic, women who'd known Khun Noi for several years, to talk with her at the brothel where she worked. We drove outside the town into lush countryside. It was early afternoon, a blazing day in orchard country famous for lychee and mangos. We took a farm road that eventually turned into a dirt track. This track led to a large orchard. We drove perhaps a kilometer through the trees, passing no one. Then we came to a clearing, which was also a parking lot. There was an outdoor beer garden under the trees. About twenty men were quietly drinking beer, sitting on rough plank benches. There was very little conversation, and our arrival seemed to spark little interest. The Mama-San (the word is used by Thais for madam) said that Khun Noi was busy with a client, and would we mind waiting?

I sat on a bench while the nurses chatted with the Mama-San, and watched the scene. Across the benches from where the men were sitting was a kind of outdoor deck. Behind this deck was a string of about 10 shacks made of bamboo and tin. Sitting on the deck were perhaps 15 young women. They were watching a Thai soap opera on a portable television. They watched the soap, the men watched them, I watched the men. Occasionally a man would make a gesture to the pimp, a young guy wearing about twelve gold chains, having made his selection. The pimp then told the girl, and she would go to her shack, to be met by the client. After a while, the scene got increasingly bizarre and uncomfortable. The men stared at the women with a kind of flat dull hunger. Country people, farmers and laborers, nonchalant but subdued. Waiting to get laid. The open erotic content of the scene, a country brothel on an ordinary day, made sex impossible not to think about. But it was the lowest common denominator of sex, as bodily function, as commodity, as urge. The women stared at the television with detachment. It was not clear, from their eyes, that they were present at all.

Khun Noi appeared, coming out of one of the shacks behind a man in his fifties, adjusting his trousers as he walked toward his car. She was tall and fair for a Thai, smiling sweetly, and elaborately polite to the nurses, who she called 'older sisters'. They held her hands. There was much laughter all around: it was an utterly natural Thai ladies' conversation.

Khun Noi was an ethnic Shan from a rural part of Thailand's Chiang Rai province. She had come here to help support her family, and had been sending money home, whenever she could, for many years. She had already built her parents a new home. She was 31, and divorced. She had one daughter, who her mother was raising. Although she worked in a fairly cheap rural brothel, she had not been trafficked – she had known what she was getting into; it was common in her home village for women to come south looking for work, and sex work was work. I liked her honesty and her dignity, but I was embarrassed for her in a way the nurses seemed not to be. When she first appeared out of the room I felt a wave of unease, even of shame. I'd been thinking, 'We're sitting here waiting for some guy to come.' It felt uncomfortable too, to be a man in this group of women, when the only reason men came here was for sex. Khun Noi seemed so gracious, so *exposed*, and all the more so for being a bright and personable woman in such a loveless place. I couldn't help but think of the nurses, their husbands, their sons, the knowledge that must be somewhere playing across their minds: he does this too – they all do it.

This is why, since the sex trade is clearly going to continue, sex workers need the protection of the law, access to medical care, and protection from debt-bondage. Sex work does not have to be slavery. ASEAN does not have to tolerate slavery or the corruption that allows slavery to continue. Trafficking will keep HIV flourishing in the region, until there is the political will to do something about it, which means reform of the police, among other large undertakings. Until such reforms come about, HIV will probably continue to have a field day in ASEAN. And women and girls from marginal communities will continue to be trafficked into the short, brutal life of sexual slavery.

Khun Noi, by the way, did agree to be in our research project, but disappeared soon after. It turned out that she was not one of the people with 'resistance' to HIV. She had used condoms consistently with her clients, and never did become infected while working in the brothel in the orchard. She stopped sex work about six months after our meeting, and the nurses told me that she came to visit them about six months after that. She had remarried, and had become HIV-infected through unprotected sex with her new husband. Condoms were for clients, not husbands.

Note

1. There are no refugee camps for the Shans along the Thai–Burmese border. If Shans come to Thailand they must find work or starve. This is not the case with the Karen, for example, 80,000 of whom live in camps along this border.

11. Military studies

Kai Kawila Royal Thai Army Camp, Chiang Mai, Thailand is the command post of the 33rd Military Circle, for the six provinces which comprise the northern section of the Thai–Burmese border, arguably Thailand's least secure. Huge old rain trees line the service roads through the expansive grounds, past orderly rows of green lorries taller than elephants. You receive crisp salutes as you pass, see army nurses in crisp white, and young men with buzz cuts, green fatigues, and shiny black boots in the fierce heat. The *taharn gain*, the conscripts, look the picture of young male health – athletic, fit, ranging from lean to brutish – marching, doing ground work, shouting out answers to shouted commands. In 1992, every tenth *taharn* in this camp had HIV infection. By 1995, half the beds in the Kai Kawila Army Hospital were reserved for AIDS care – beds that are now nearly always used. The men dying here are very young, many in their early 20s. It takes a visit to the hospital to see how much the image of male vigor displayed on the marching ground is an illusion. This is the army of a smallish country at peace with itself, its neighbors, and the wider world, and yet the death rate here has been higher than in many spectacular battles. To lose a tenth of something is to have it decimated. Decimation is happening here, and not a shot has been fired.

Addressing an audience of high-ranking military officers from a friendly foreign state on the subject of the sexual behavior and drug- and alcohol-using activities of their soldiers can be tricky. You have to try to read your listeners' faces, to see what they already know, and how ready they are to face new information, to make tough choices. When I first came to Thailand we had a good deal of information on hand (from an earlier military study) to say that sex with another man raised the risk of a Thai soldier being HIV-positive from one in eight to one in five. This could only mean unprotected

140

anal intercourse, and that the men engaging in it were not using condoms. We suggested to the officers that we needed to include safer anal sex practices for both homosexuals and heterosexuals in all the military HIV-prevention programs. I know that my voice was steady: I could hear it via the microphone in the cold conference room, but my hands were shaking as I made this proposal. The room, however, was all nods and smiles: 'Yes, we will do that. Next point please.' And they did. During the Clinton débâcle over gays in the military, and the subsequent adoption of the 'Don't ask, don't tell' policy, the Thai head of the Joint Chiefs of Staff, General Wimol, was asked if gays would be allow to serve in the Thai Military. He answered that the Thai Military had always had homosexuals, that many had served with distinction, and that there was no need for a change in policy. Next point please. (What alarms Americans, given the very real threats to peace and stability in the world, is peculiar. We think ourselves practical and Asians mystical, but we respond most powerfully not to information but to symbols: burning flags; sodomy on ships; school prayer; the sexual continence, or lack thereof, of our leaders.)

It seems only natural that HIV should affect armies more than civilians. Most soldiers, obviously, are young men. In Burma the starting age is 15; in Thailand 21; in the Khmer Rouge insurgency, perhaps 12 or 13. These are young men far from home, family, and friends. They are largely the rural and urban poor, with little or moderate education and limited work experience. Once conscripted, alone and under intense pressure, they seek support from all-male groups, looking for buddies, mates, best friends. We know that this is true from well-conducted studies of the behavior of soldiers, and also from the best war writing: from Hemingway, James Jones, Wilfred Owen, Homer, and Thucydides. Young soldiers drink together; they blow off steam; they go whoring together – as much to be together as to be with a woman. Far from wives and girlfriends, they find cheap brothels close to their bases. The relationship between soldiers and sex workers is as old as war itself; it is for this reason that military medicine has had to concern itself with sexually spread infections in the past, and with HIV now.

Only a handful of pharmaceutical manufacturers are working on HIV vaccines. With few exceptions (currently three), most of the vaccines under development are aimed at only one subtype of HIV:

subtype B, present in the US, Western Europe, and Australia. A vaccine that worked against this subtype might or might not protect against any of the other subtypes. For the bulk of the potential paying market, this may not matter very much. For most people in the world, who live where other subtypes predominate (Africa, Asia) this limitation may well mean that the HIV vaccines under development will protect neither them nor their children. And, it need hardly be said, these are the great majority of people who are likely to get HIV, though not the B subtype. There is a desperate lack of research activity into the viruses affecting most of the world; there is no major vaccine manufacturer working on a vaccine that might be of use in Africa, where one is perhaps most needed, and where non-vaccine interventions have had the least success. This gap has been partly filled by the US Army, and the Walter Reed Army Institute for Research (WRAIR), among others. This is simply because the American soldier is as likely to have sex with a prostitute in Bangkok as in Las Vegas, and is potentially vulnerable to exposure to every HIV subtype known (and some, undoubtedly, as yet unknown). WRAIR has been a leader in HIV research, vaccine research, and vaccine development for the non-B subtypes of HIV. This has also meant that WRAIR has had to establish research partnerships outside the US. Its relationship with Thai Army medical researchers goes back 30 years. Thailand has had US-military-supported medical research facilities since then. It is a close, productive relationship, though one not easily grasped by those outside the field. (The most recent success of this collaboration has been the development of a vaccine against hepatitis A, the field trials of which were conducted in Thailand, where the disease is common and a significant problem in facilities like schools and nurseries.)

Many American civilians (and I include myself) have lingering negative associations with our military and its overseas exploits. We associate the medical/scientific activities of the US military with Agent Orange, napalm and toxic defoliants, and with atmospheric testing of atomic weapons in the presence of uninformed soldiers. We have seen the grainy black and white footage from the Nevada test site, with soldiers lined up in the killing wind. We suspect that we are not told the whole truth about the research activities of the Pentagon. We are not alone in these anxieties: it is still widely believed in the Caribbean and in Africa, as well as among American blacks, for example, that HIV is a US germ-warfare experiment gone awry. (There are several versions of this story, involving an attempt to wipe out the pigs of Castro's Cuba with a CIA-created virus tested first in Haiti, or in Africa. This, interestingly, turned out to have been a KGB disinformation campaign against the Reagan administration, revealed when the USSR crumbled and Kremlin documents describing the campaign were declassified.) What is striking about working with the WRAIR group, at least those involved in HIV research -- the only ones I know well -- is how far their intentions are from such conspiracies. As a group, they are, if anything, more idealistic and impassioned than the civilian research sector. WRAIR's limitations have not, by and large, been a lack of concern or a resistance to working with HIV, as much as budgetary restraints imposed by the Federal Office of Management and Budget (OMB). WRAIR scientists have used sympathetic members of Congress to beef up their HIV budgets for years, performing a rearguard action around the Federal bureaucrats whose bottom line has been budget-reduction, not an HIV vaccine that would work against exotic forms of the virus. The political football in this struggle – that of gay men and women serving in the US Armed Forces[1] – has been something of a side issue as far as WRAIR's research program has been concerned.

Because the AIDS epidemic has been so closely connected to homosexuality in the US, military and civilian sectors alike have had to confront their own institutional homophobia, and that of Congress, the electorate, and the vocal Christian Right. This has been a complex and emotional interaction, fraught with weak, ideological thinking, though it could be argued that the military has done a better job of caring for its infected members than many civilian sectors. Some of this is due to the pioneering work of Dr Robert Redfield, the WRAIR researcher who first described heterosexual transmission of HIV among US servicemen with a history of prostitute use. This was a key contribution: until Redfield's work (it seems incredible now, given what has happened in Africa and Asia, where HIV is overwhelmingly a disease of heterosexuals) being HIV-infected was virtually tantamount to being classed as a hemophiliac, an injecting drug user, or a homosexual man – all grounds for exclusion from the armed forces. After Redfield's landmark paper, one could simply be an unlucky heterosexual. It was General Phil Russell, the head of WRAIR's vaccine division in the mid 1980s, who made another important contribution: he argued that the men and women with HIV in the US armed forces were a potentially valuable group for research on HIV/AIDS. They were eligible for veterans' benefits, and could be followed long-term. Since the military had already mandated regular HIV testing for all members, all HIV-infected personnel could be included in these studies, if they agreed. And agreement has been close to 100%, generating some important insights into the long-term survival of people with AIDS while allowing HIV-infected personnel to maintain non-combat duties, dignity, and veterans' benefits. It was a conservative Christian member of the House of Representatives – Dannenmeyer of California – who attempted, against the wishes of the military, to force people with HIV and AIDS out of the armed forces, by means of a pointless, punitive Bill which President Clinton, in an act of calculated cowardice, signed into law in 1996. It is currently being challenged in the courts; the administration clearly knew in advance that this would occur, as it is flagrantly unconstitutional, and violates the Americans with Disabilities Act, made law by President Bush, which includes HIV/AIDS as a disability.

Encouragingly, rates of new HIV infection in the US military have been relatively low, low enough for preventive studies, such as HIV-vaccine trials, to have become virtually impossible. So few new infections happen each year that it would take decades, and cost tens of millions of dollars, to find an HIV vaccine using the army as a study population. Enter Thailand, a close US ally, with a large, very high-risk military, high rates of new infection, and a marked eagerness to look for new solutions.

The problem with the Thai army is that it, too, is a poor population for HIV-vaccine studies. Thai conscripts serve only two years, and are difficult to follow thereafter. As they are not volunteers, research on this group is not ethically straightforward. Most crucially, rates of new HIV infection in this group, as we have seen, fell off dramatically once preventive measures had been put in place. By the time an HIV vaccine including antigens against the Thai virus was close to testing, epidemic rates of new infections among Thai soldiers had largely passed. This is why the WRAIR group has been forced to go farther afield, looking at Thai civilians attending STD clinics, at factory workers, at pregnant women, and considering other countries in the region. There have been some questions raised as to why the military should be funding research in civilian sectors. Their mandate however, has been clear: to protect the American soldier through the development of a preventive vaccine, and there is currently no other way to do this than through expanding the research base.

Some countries, however, are not being considered, most notably Burma. The US military has, to its credit (this is a personal opinion) steadfastly refused to deal with the SLORC. Burma's army actually reports comparatively low rates of HIV infection – less than 2% in 1994 – but these data cannot be taken at face value. The Burmese army is young: with conscription beginning at 15, it is an army partially composed of children and adolescents, who may not have begun risk behaviors. And, clearly, information on the SLORC which they themselves are willing to divulge is heavily censored. One study of HIV risks among men in the Burmese military has been reported, though not, as yet, published in full. Risk behaviors were common, and included sex with other men (7.4%), extra-marital sex (13%), sex with CSWs (37.3%) and inconsistent or absent condom use (96.6%). The prevalence of syphilis was slightly higher than that of HIV, at 2.5%. Taken together, these risks and the syphilis finding make the very low reported prevalence of HIV look even less real. There are some differences between the civilian and military health sectors in Burma that may also be of importance. The military has the resources to do a better job of screening blood, to use disposable injection equipment, and to practice safer surgery and medical procedures in general, at least in the cities and at major military installations. What actually occurs is, as always in Burma, unknown. We do know that donations of medical equipment, drugs, and condoms intended for the civilians of Burma have largely been funneled toward the military. And it was the military medical corps which did the behavioral study quoted here, a rare example of the kind of research Burma desperately needs to understand the health and behavior of its people.

The Lao military, not surprisingly, is another unknown. One encouraging sign, however, has been a series of discreet meetings between Lao and Thai military medical staff. In a perfect world, the Lao authorities would be able to learn from their Thai neighbors, and initiate prevention soon. The Cambodian military has been somewhat more open; they are facing disaster. Surveys among Khmer soldiers on the Thai–Cambodian frontier found that about 30% of the Khmer troops were HIV-infected. While these data are also somewhat dubious, and the samples small, there is clearly a huge problem. But this is only what we know of the national army; the Khmer Rouge army remains an information black hole.

The Khmer Rouge is, of course, not the only insurgent force in Southeast Asia. Burma has more than 15 ethnic insurgencies, Laos at least one, the Philippines several, including ethnic, communist, and Muslim insurgencies. India probably leads this field in Asia: there are more than fifteen insurgencies in the northeastern states alone (including Manipur, Mizoram, Tripura, Assam, Nagaland, Arunachal Pradesh, and Meghalaya) as well as in Kashmir. What health programs there are for the young men (and women) in these struggles tend to be rudimentary at best; these populations are not small, and HIV is undoubtedly circulating among some of them. These groups, like the Burmese insurgents and the Khmer Rouge, are involved in 'low-intensity' chronic civil wars, the kind of military and political struggles that so often involve civilians, women and children, and that blur the distinctions between military and civilian populations. They are extraordinarily difficult populations to reach for assistance of any kind – medical, educational, or preventive. And they are terribly vulnerable to disease. A Burmese soldier in the one armed group fighting for democracy told me that '. . . our first enemy is malaria; our second is leeches; SLORC is third.' HIV should probably be on the list as well, though where in the hierarchy of suffering is unlikely to be known for years to come.

Note

1. For a thorough investigation of this saga, see Randy Shilts's *Conduct Unbecoming: Gays & Lesbians in the U.S. Military* (St. Martins Press, New York, 1993).

12. Chasing the dragon: heroin and AIDS

When a man walks hand in hand with the thirst of craving, he will wander from birth to birth, now here, now there, and with never an end in sight.

The Sutta Nipata

Dr Ken Nelson has studied the relationships between injecting drug use and HIV since the early days of the epidemic in the US. He came to Johns Hopkins from the University of Illinois, after a distinguished career as an infectious-disease physician and epidemiologist, to pursue HIV work. Ken has done medical research in Thailand for more than 20 years, initially on rabies, then on leprosy; he was an American epidemiologist who knew Thailand intimately before HIV arrived. Since then, he has never wavered from an intense focus on mitigating what he knew, by 1991, was going to be a disaster. He brought me to Thailand in 1992, and it was largely through his contacts, and the respect in which he is held by Thai scientists, that we were able to move expeditiously into HIV-prevention research in Chiang Mai.

In Baltimore, Ken had been working for several years with gay men and injecting addicts (most injectors in Baltimore use 'speedball', heroin and cocaine in the same syringe). A Johns Hopkins colleague, Dr David Vlahov, had developed the ALIVE study, a large, long-term follow-up program for nearly 3,000 Baltimore drug users. Ken had an elegant idea in the late 1980s, when about 5% of addicts per year were becoming newly HIV-infected despite intensive education, counseling, and freely available drug treatment. He thought an essential question could be evaluated among the ALIVE participants. While rates of new HIV infection were falling among gay men, and had fallen to almost zero among hemophiliacs and transfusion recipients in the US, inner-city addicts like those in Baltimore continued to be infected at a high, steady rate. One of the few groups of people in the US with ready access to sterile needles are diabetics dependent on insulin. Since diabetics typically need daily injections of insulin, they get standing prescriptions for needles along with their medication. Ken's idea was to compare the HIV rate among diabetic heroin addicts with those who were not diabetic. The result: addicts with diabetes were strikingly less likely to be HIV-infected than those without the disease. Why? They had legal access to clean needles and knew how to use them. These findings were published in the *Journal of the American Medical Association* in October 1991. The simplicity of this study, and the elegance of its findings, support a conclusion both logical, and, in the American political climate, radical. If addicts had access to clean needles, HIV rates could be reduced.

Narcotics Anonymous (NA), a national support group based on the tradition of Alcoholics Anonymous, defines addiction as an illness. NA maintains that addicts are ill, not criminal. If this is the case, should addicts be treated like other persons in need of clean syringes, such as diabetics, and be allowed prescriptions? This proposition falls under the rubric of harm reduction; while getting off drugs is the ideal in the long term, harm-reduction strategies seek to reduce those complications of drug use amenable to change, such as HIV infection. Assisting addicts to reduce needle-sharing is harm-reduction, as is needle exchange, another seemingly simple approach to reducing HIV spread among addicts: you offer users new needles in exchange for used ones. Dirty needles are taken out of circulation, and addicts have less need to share, since the exchange solves their chronic shortage problem. This is practical, simple, effective, and virtually impossible to implement in the United States.

In the land of 'Just Say No', harm-reduction strategies have proven politically problematic. The arguments against needle-exchange programs have invariably resorted to a handful of unproven, but telling, assumptions: providing needles condones drug use; it promotes drug use; it encourages addicts to continue using drugs, since using is made safer. None of these assumptions is supported by hard evidence, yet the debate around these simplistic notions has been classically American in its passion and intensity. The evidence suggests, if anything, that addicts in exchange programs are more likely to enter drug treatment, since the exchange programs become points of contact between otherwise isolated addicts and the health-care system. Needle exchanges can build trust, open lines of communication, and help build bridges to marginal communities. They can help addicts get into treatment programs. But, like frank sex education in schools, or contraceptive services for sexually active youth, the idea of harm reduction through needle exchange has been seen less as a necessary health intervention than as a moral threat. It took five years for Baltimore to begin a needle-exchange program after the publication of Ken's findings, years in which several thousand people needlessly became infected with HIV.

It has been left to activists in the US to mount needle-exchange programs in the great majority of communities where government and public health bodies have refused to do so. In most States, such programs are illegal, underground and under-funded. The same situation exists in another country where moralistic (and religious) responses to HIV have made harm reduction a contentious political issue – Malaysia. An underground needle exchange has operated in Malaysia on and off for several years. The government, so far, has turned a blind eye to the exchange. They have recognized its utility, but have been unable politically to support it. As with public health officials in the US, everybody knows it is the right thing to do, and that the scientific evidence is compelling, but harm reduction stands in sharp contrast to the government policy of 'eradication' of drug use.

What do an Islamic nationalist party and the US Democratic and Republican parties have in common? Ideological stances that have led to the inability to respond to science with coherent public policy, and vocal fundamentalist minorities who have been successful in compelling governments to shape laws and policies in accordance with their moral and religious dictates. Public health and its practitioners have had mixed results in countering these groups. We have been naive, at best, in thinking that if we did our part well (research, publications, presentations to political bodies), logical outcomes in public policy would follow. But time and again, in Malaysia, and in the US, irrational, unsound, and poorly informed policies have been implemented, while those backed by solid data have languished. We have been much less activist in orientation than the anti-scientific fundamentalists, and they have been more successful in shaping policy.

Are there other examples of this? The ban on HIV-infected persons traveling to the United States was meant to 'protect' Americans from HIV. It was signed into law when the US already had more than a million cases, more than all of Europe. This ban applied not only to immigration, which might be a more complex issue, and which might actually be enforceable (since physical examinations and blood tests are routinely done on prospective immigrants); just entering the US is illegal for any HIV-positive person. It was this restriction that forced Harvard University to host the 1991 International AIDS Meeting in Amsterdam instead of Boston: an international embarrassment for the Bush administration. This law is still in effect. It has had no discernible effect on the US epidemic, which anyone looking at the epidemiology of HIV could have predicted, but it has certainly supported other governments who have also wished to restrict the freedom of people with AIDS.

If we look carefully at the pattern of HIV epidemics in Southeast Asia, the first group to undergo the rapid phase of HIV spread in Thailand, Burma, Yunnan, and Malaysia were injecting users. In all four cases, needle sharing was the key behavior underlying these bursts. Once several thousand addicts were infected, the spread to non-addict populations in Thailand and Burma, at least, was rapid and pervasive. This pattern suggests that prevention of early HIV spread among addicts could be crucial for prevention of national epidemics in countries with significant numbers of injecting drug users. This possibility makes harm reduction for addicts a priority. Tragically, it has not proven to be any more politically feasible in Asia than in the US. Even Thailand, the acknowledged regional leader in prevention, is only now considering needle exchange (under Dr Chawalit).

The Northern Drug Dependency Treatment Center (NDDTC) is a Thai government facility for the treatment of drug addiction. It is in Mae Rim, a mixed suburban and farming district to the north of Chiang Mai, close to San Sai and Doi Saket, where the widows' group is active. Several kilometers down a country road, beside a Buddhist temple and a small branch of the Ping river, the NDDTC is in an idyllic place. The Director, Dr Jaroon Juttiwutikarn, is a Thai psychiatrist and a specialist in the treatment of substance abuse. The program at NDDTC reflects Dr Jaroon's humane, realistic approach to drug treatment, as well as the Thai government's commitment to funding treatment programs adequately. The basic concept is that of Narcotics Anonymous: addicts are people with an illness who need treatment, not criminals deserving punishment. Admission is voluntary and addicts can leave at any time. Heroin addicts are treated with methadone on a tapering dose, opium addicts with tincture of opium, in both cases to relieve the physical symptoms of withdrawal, which can be excruciating. (Detoxification without these treatments is 'cold turkey', an expression derived from the chills of withdrawal, and the pilo-erection – body hair literally standing on end – which gives the withdrawing addicts' limbs the look of turkey skin, or gooseflesh.) The program takes three weeks, though addicts can stay longer (up to a year) if they feel the need. In addition to the detox medications, addicts get counseling and health checks; it is a quiet, supportive environment in which to break out of the cycle of addiction. Meditation classes are regularly given by visiting Buddhist monks. There is also Thai traditional therapy. The center's gardens grow Thai medicinal herbs, which are used in a herbal sauna. After the first week of detox in a hospital-like ward, the addicts begin these herbal saunas, and also receive therapeutic massage. These traditional therapies are used to alleviate the physical symptoms of withdrawal, but also to return a sense of well-being and wholeness to people who may have neglected their physical selves for years.

The NDDTC is a beautiful place, and a hopeful one. While treatment failures are common (only about 15% of addicts stay permanently drug-free after one admission), and many addicts may be admitted several times for detox before they are finally free, the men and women (and children) who come to NDDTC are treated with dignity, concern, and compassion. Since drug treatment in Laos, Burma, and Malaysia is only cold turkey, and in all three countries is on a criminal, not a medical, model, a significant percentage of patients come from these countries. With the desire to get off drugs, and fear of their own countries' programs, addicts risk arrest to get to Thailand for treatment. The Thai government accepts whoever walks into NDDTC. The first time I went I met a young Canadian girl, half-way through the program, slowly and shakily coming back to life.

While most patients at NDDTC are Thai nationals, only half are ethnic Thais. The other half are tribal people: Hmong, Akha, Lisu, Lahu, Karen, Yao. The two groups are strikingly different. Nearly all the ethnic Thais are men, most are young, and almost all are heroin addicts, either injectors or men who 'chase the dragon' – heroin smokers. The tribal people are much more heterogenous: men, women and children are represented. Addicted families come for treatment together. The majority are opium smokers, though heroin use is increasing among some groups. Because opiates are passed through the breast milk of nursing mothers, some of the addicts from these tribal groups are babies. When their mothers stop using, they too go into withdrawal. At NDDTC they are given oral tincture of opium in pediatric doses to ease their suffering. It is an extraordinary sight: tribal women with their babies strapped to their backs walking in groups around the grounds; village women, who are used to meeting at wells, lining up for their daily doses of detox.

The Thais and tribal peoples at NDDTC have very different HIV rates: about half the Thais are HIV-positive; among the hill tribes, the rate is only about 8%. Some of the difference may be due to the Thais being likely to be needle users, and the tribal peoples to be smokers. But some of it may be due to other factors, such as sexual risks. An unknown percentage of the Thai addicts have sold sex to support their habits, a dual risk that is only too common in the West.

Will any of Thailand's neighbors follow her lead in the humane treatment of addicts? Burma and Laos, arguably, do not have the resources for treatment centers as well funded as the Thai national ones. Malaysia's program, with its mandatory two years' incarceration, is already many times more expensive, and its success rate no better, if not worse. China also has mandatory drug treatment: it is also cold turkey only, and also has a low success rate. What limits these national responses is largely ideology, rather than science or money. In this regard, the Thais also have yet to take two further steps that men like Dr Jaroon know could help reduce the terrible burden of HIV among Thai addicts. One is needle exchange, which started in Chiang Mai only in 1996; the other is a controversial program called methadone maintenance.

Methadone is a synthetic morphine derivative related to opium, heroin, and morphine. It is just as addicting as its sister compounds, if not more so. But it has several features which have long made it the drug of choice for detoxification: it is given orally, so it frees addicts from needle use; it can manage the opiate craving which drives users back to heroin or opium (scientific evidence suggests methadone may work by saturating the opiate receptors in the brain, thereby reducing the craving for opiates); and it is a legal, prescription drug, which doctors can give to patients. This is something of a historical accident, and there are probably better agents for detox than powerfully addicting methadone, but it is legal, so it continues to be used. The standard therapy in Thailand, which is a matter of national policy, is methadone taper: the dose of methadone is tapered off over several months till the addict is 'drug free'. The problem is the craving. Each addict has his or her own level of methadone above which they are craving-free, but below which they start to crave, withdraw, and suffer. Some make it, but many use heroin again, usually in combination with the insufficient methadone dose, to handle the hunger. By the time addicts are tapered completely off methadone, they are often back on their old dose of heroin, and the detox cycle begins all over again. Methadone maintenance accepts that some addicts are not going to lose their craving, at least in the short term, and that going back to heroin use means going back to needle use, and sharing – the spiral of disease risk. Methadone maintenance is another form of harm reduction: let the addicts set their own level of methadone such that they don't need heroin, and let them stay at that dose at long as they need it, to keep them clear of the need for needles, for life, if necessary. (Remember that about half of northern Thai heroin addicts are HIV-infected already, so keeping these men off heroin is essential to protect new addicts from HIV – it is already too late for many long-term users.)

Methadone maintenance was tried once in Bangkok among addicts, in a pilot project done by the Bangkok Metropolitan Authority (BMA) in 1991. While the BMA didn't look at the effect of the therapy on HIV rates, they did look at maintenance in terms of addicts remaining in follow-up and staying off heroin. By those criteria it was an unmitigated success; addicts tapered completely off methadone were much less likely to stay in treatment, and much more likely to go back to heroin use. But, as so often has been the case with AIDS, political considerations delayed the translation of these research findings into public health policy, in this case by at least five years. Why? The Thai Ministry of Social Welfare, which oversees drug treatment programs, refused to change their policy from taper to maintenance. Taper means you are getting people 'off drugs'; it is politically attractive, even if it usually fails. Maintenance means you accept that some people are not going to get free of opiate addiction, but can at least be treated to prevent needle-use relapses. It works, and there is evidence to show that it works, but it is politically 'sensitive', as Dr Jaroon explained to me, too sensitive to implement even in the midst of an epidemic of a new, fatal virus spread through needle sharing.

Why should human frailty be so hard for political bodies to accept? Why are we so tempted by absolutist and simplistic models of human behavior that repeatedly fail to achieve their stated goals? One would think, given the track record of politicians in any country, that they would be the group most eager to embrace forgiveness of human frailty. We look so hard for 'cures', for the magic bullets that will solve complex social and medical problems: a vaccine to protect against HIV, new therapies for AIDS care. But simple steps such as giving addicts prescriptions for needles, implementing needle exchanges, offering methadone maintenance programs, remain beyond our reach. Compared to the cost and difficulty of AIDS treatment, these are cheap and easy. Preventing HIV spread among addicts might even prevent national HIV epidemics in some countries. But supporting such programs might open a politician to charges of being 'soft' on drugs, and anything is better than that, including being 'soft' on AIDS.

13. Tribes: the virus that kills the gods

[I]t is clear that tribal vulnerability to HIV must be placed within the macro context – national, regional, and global – of changed commercial routes, the entry of urban-based governments and entrepreneurs into the hills, and the migration of hill people into urban centres, as well as the political and economic chaos in neighboring Burma which helps to foster the thriving illicit economy.

'Vulnerability to HIV Infection Among Three Hill Tribes in Northern Thailand' (Kammerer et al., 1995)

The dominant peoples of Southeast Asia have always been lowlanders of the irrigated plains and river valleys: the Thais, Burmans, Khmers, Vietnamese. The hills and mountains of the region, tail-end spires of the Himalayan range, have been home to very different peoples. The highland ethnic minorities of Indochina number in the hundreds, and are found in every country of the region. They are a heterogenous array of peoples, clans, languages, faiths, and ethnicities. These groups include the indigenous headhunting Wa, the stone age 'spirits of the yellow leaves', and the literate Yao, who practice a mystical form of Taoism and venerate the Chinese poet-sage, Lao Tzu. Some, like the nomadic Akha of Yunnan, Burma, and northern Thailand, are animists, though the Akha language is a dialect of Tibetan. Others, like the Hmong of Laos, China, and Vietnam, once had a kingdom of their own, but lost it to Han Chinese, and have been wandering, like the Hebrews, ever since. Relations between highlanders and lowlanders have been a constant theme in the history of the region, often tumultuous, and seldom to the benefit of these tribal peoples.

The great majority of highland communities continue to survive on subsistence agriculture. Slash-and-burn, or swidden, farming techniques are widespread. Prosperity is not. The highlanders lag in education, in health measures such as infant mortality and life expectancy, in literacy, and in political clout. They are a tremendously diverse group in terms of HIV/AIDS risks and rates. Some, like the ethnic Karen in Thailand, have thus far been apparently spared epidemic spread of HIV. Others, like the Wa, the Lahu, and the Kachin of Burma and China, and the Akha in northern Thailand, are likely to be severely affected. Reaching these peoples has not been a priority of most governments in the region. The Shans are still at war with the Burmans; the Hmong and Yao in Laos with the lowland Lao; the Mizos, Manipuris, Nagas, and Assamese are still at war with India, and often with each other. Even where there is peace, the challenges are immense, not only because languages and dialects often isolate the highlanders from majority populations, but also because their understanding of disease and health are often pre-scientific, magical, and unstudied.

The Lahus in Burma are one such group. They are nomadic people from the Tibetan plateau, who have gradually moved south over several centuries. The first Lahu village in Thailand was founded in the 1940s, but they have been in Burma much longer. Burmese is also a Tibeto-Burman language, but is unintelligible to the Lahu. In Burma they have the misfortune to be geographically isolated between the warring Shans, Wa, and SLORC, and are themselves divided into several different groups, including the Red and the Black Lahu clans. (These two groups have formed a political alliance, the Lahu Democratic Front.) When AIDS education materials first came to the Lahu, these were in the form of pamphlets and posters in Burmese. The pamphlets warned that AIDS was 'nat thi', meaning incurable. Nats are the Burmese folk deities, the local gods. The Lahu interpretation was that AIDS could 'kill nats', that this new disease, which the Burmans were so afraid of, killed both men and gods. And this is how HIV was first known among them. What happens to a Lahu woman who comes home after sex work in Thailand, carrying a virus fatal to the local spirits?

As most Lahu in Burma are illiterate, HIV education has to be done through oral media: radio, video, cassettes, talking. SLORC has recently taken to jamming the uncensored radio broadcasts that once reached the mountains of the Lahu, limiting the effectiveness of this medium for mass education. One solution has come from an unexpected quarter: Lahu sex workers in Chiang Mai. With NGO assistance, a group of Lahu women have made a series of HIV educational cassettes, and these have been distributed through trading networks in the Lahus' remote homeland. These tapes explain not only what HIV is, and how it can be prevented, but also how trafficking works, what a woman can expect if she comes through this route to Thailand, how to use a telephone and what numbers to call if she comes to Thailand and needs help. Because so many tribal groups have had women trafficked to Thailand, such programs, if the groups themselves could accept assistance from 'broken women', could have a significant impact in Burma. At present, there are few other such programs.

I met one of the Lahu leaders in August 1996, and had a frank discussion about the situation in Burma. His principal concerns were three: injections from untrained practitioners (who he called, charmingly, 'quacks'); heroin use among Lahu men, which he felt was on the increase; and the trafficking of Lahu women and girls. Did he think condom use could be accepted by Lahu men, or at least those men with wives who had been sex workers? Yes, he said, he thought so, but he himself had never seen a condom. What was it, exactly? Did I happen to have one?

We know that the bulk of China's documented HIV cases are among highland minority peoples; fully 60% of the national total of infections have been identified in Kachins, Wa, and Dai. In Burma it is clear that highland groups are as heavily affected by HIV as the Burmans. In Thailand one systematic survey of HIV has been done among hill-tribe groups: a 1994–95 survey of nine minorities, carried out by the Thai Red Cross in collaboration with our group. What we found was that HIV rates varied tremendously between groups, from zero cases among the Karen, to 9% of all adults among the Shans. The aggregated rate in adults aged 15–45 was 2.1%, lower than the Thai rate in the northern region, but higher than the Thai national average. Sexual behavior, social norms, and attitudes toward HIV all varied just as strikingly; these groups are as different from each other as the Irish are from the Yoruba. But one thing did not differ greatly, and this was the risk factor associated with being HIV-positive. There was really only one risk, and it superseded ethnicity: for women, having been a worker in the sex industry; for men, having been a patron. In our study at least, tribal people with HIV were those who had been touched by the sex trade in the lowlands. We found HIV-infected women in seven of the nine ethnic groups studied, but infected men in only three of the nine. The two groups where no cases were found, the Karen and the Pa-long, police their own communities and do not allow trafficking. Several Karen communities are known to shoot brothel traffickers on sight. This may not be a prevention strategy that one would like to see spread, but it cannot be called a failure.

My Thai colleagues and I have presented the findings you have just read many times in Thailand, to academic audiences, medical groups, and the government. Each time we've done so the results have been met with disbelief. The usual assumption is that the tribal groups have much higher rates than the Thais, due to their habits of 'free sex', their loose morals, poor hygiene, and heavy heroin use. That the major risk for HIV among minority peoples should be the Thai sex industry seems incredible to Thai audiences. But the evidence is fairly compelling. If local spread were the root cause, we would expect to see what is found in most other communities: either equal rates among men and women, or higher rates among men – not four ethnic groups where all HIV-positives were women and none men. But the highlanders are a classic example of the 'other', the 'outsider', to lowland majorities, and HIV comes from the other, not the self.

HIV prevention for these communities in Thailand is clearly going to require a focus on trafficking. In China, heroin use will be key. For the ethnic minorities in Burma, both heroin use and trafficking are going to have to be addressed, and both will be extraordinarily difficult to remedy under the SLORC regime. For the hill tribes in Burma, the prognosis is painfully poor. Of the highlanders in Vietnam, Laos, and Cambodia, little can be said as so little is known. The one exception, perhaps, is the Hmong of Laos, who have a long, complex history of exchange with the outside world, who have been known, even if they are now abandoned and forgotten.

Diaspora: The fate of the Hmong

The domino theory of communist expansion has been fairly thoroughly discredited. It now seems as dated and wrong-headed as the Hollywood blacklist, or the 'red' in Red China. The media, with their seemingly unconscious Western bias, routinely talk about the 'fall of communism'. We find ourselves saying 'now that the Cold War is over', just as we stumble over leaving out 'the' when we say Ukraine. But while the Czechs race toward Europe and the many new -stans to Islam, China, Vietnam, and Laos are still ruled by geriatric politburos. The men who led the Communist revolutions of these neighbors are very much in power. The Hmong people of Laos really were a domino that fell to the communists. They paid the heaviest price you can pay for their resistance to the Viet Cong-supported takeover of Laos: defeat, impoverishment, loss of their native lands, slaughter, and exile.

The Hmong are a proud, fierce people. Accounts by the French and Americans who fought with them are strikingly consistent in their respect for these small, tough, mountain people. It took nine years of war and the invasion of over 70,000 Vietnamese troops to drive the Hmong off their mountains in Laos, so fierce was their resistance. More than 100,000 Hmong from those mountains have been resettled in the US, where the rich, ancient Hmong tribal culture is a poor preparation for immigrant success. Self-sufficient people of the limestone crags, slash-and-burn farmers, hunters and trappers, they now must survive on the outskirts of Los Angeles, San Diego, and Minneapolis.

No one knows how many thousands of Hmong were killed during the long wars in which they fought beside two losers, the French and the Americans. (The French called them *montagnards*, and used them as scouts. The US used them as a proxy army against Vietnam.) The real slaughter came later, after the capture of Vientiane, when the communists took their revenge with the simple slogan, 'wipe them out'. Perhaps half the Hmong population was killed in the ensuing genocide (there is no other word). Those who managed to escape to Thailand faced lives of poverty and despair in crowded camps. Unused to lowland conditions, to overcrowding and inactivity, many died. The lucky families got out, to the US, Australia, or France. The rest remained in Thailand until 1993, when the Thais initiated a policy of forced repatriation to Laos. More than 16,000 have been sent back since then. This late chapter in the saga of the Hmong has been almost totally ignored by the world's media.

The UN High Commissioner for Refugees is supposed to be overseeing the Hmong *refoulement*, but rights monitors have not been given permission to go beyond Vientiane, and that is not where the

Hmong are. It is not at all clear what is happening in the mountain-ous interior of Laos. The people who slaughtered the Hmong are still in power: not just the same party or government, but the same men who ordered and carried out the massacres. I had been told that Laos was quiet, and it was portrayed that way in the media. In Vientiane we heard rumors of fighting and insurgency in the interior, but these were unsubstantiated.

On a river journey from the Thai border to Luang Prabang, we passed several new villages of Hmong recently sent back to Laos. These riverine areas were never Hmong lands in the past. Their homeland is the mountains surrounding the Plain of Jars, the scene of their great defeat. In Luang Prabang itself, the Hmong were nowhere to be seen. On the last day of my stay I met two men on the street who had the classic stocky build and broad, high foreheads of the Hmong. The older man, about 30, asked me in English where I was from. When I said 'America' his face lit up, and so I knew he was Hmong, not Lao. We went for a walk; he was furtive, checking all directions as we went. I asked him how things were for him, now, in Laos.

'It is very bad for the Hmong. I cannot work, we have no way to make a living. Two years ago my family and I were sent back here from Chiang Khong, in Thailand. We did not like Thailand but at least we were safe there. My family is in the mountains now, some days' walking from here. I will take you if you want to see. This Lao government is very bad to us. We are forced to fight again.'

'Is there fighting now?'

'Yes, fighting. But we are alone. No one is with us.'

I promised him I would try and return, would talk to journalist friends, to try and generate some interest in their plight. He gave me his name and address and we said goodbye.

That night, when I came back from dinner, he and several more Hmong were waiting outside the hotel gate. They wanted to share my room, as they had no place to stay. But it seemed unsafe for them; the hotel was government-run; officials from Vientiane were staying there, and five Hmong men would be fairly obvious in my single room. We walked through the night streets together for a while. Their belief in the Americans was moving, but also tragic. How was I to tell them that we were most unlikely to come back and assist with their current troubles?

Soon after this meeting, a young Lao man, keeping a safe distance but always there, followed me wherever I went. Having spoken with my new Hmong friends, I had acquired a tail. This fellow appeared at the airport the next morning, as I got ready to fly back to Huai Sai on a Lao Aviation biplane. He managed to sit next to me on the flight, and I noticed he was carrying no luggage, in stark contrast to all the other Laos, who were loaded with bags, stacks of French bread, whole banana bunches. He was met by three army officers on the tarmac; I made one more round of police checks, and was allowed to leave. A bad Graham Greene sequence, but also a reminder of how tightly controlled and mistrusted the Hmong remain.

I contacted several journalists on my return to Thailand. Two or three had already heard that there was fighting again between the Hmong and the Lao, but no one was interested in covering the story. 'It's just a drug war,' said one, 'nothing political is happening there.'

The Hmong in Laos had always grown opium for medicinal use, and for the aches and pains of old age, for which it was especially reserved. Because of Laos' isolation, high mountains, and the unnavigable stretches of the Mekong as it moves south through the country, the French saw little hope of developing Laos for the lucrative plantations they had already established in Cochin. Their policy in Laos was to impose a yearly 'head tax' on all adults, and to collect this in silver. The Hmong had nothing to sell but opium, and this the French accepted. So began the long history of the Hmong as opium growers.

The Hmong in Thailand were also opium farmers, until the Thai government policy of crop substitution reached their highland homes. Some have succeeded in growing cut flowers or fruit, and in trading. But the loss of opium revenues has had an economic impact, and an impact on HIV as well. There is some evidence that as opium became unavailable for the Hmong, users switched to chasing the dragon or injecting heroin. Striking correlations have been shown by researchers at Chiang Mai University, and by the Center for AIDS Prevention Studies (CAPS) in San Francisco, of the simultaneous rise in heroin use with the decline in opium smoking. Opium the Hmong grew, heroin they must buy. And so the trafficking of Hmong girls increased as well, as addicted fathers sold their daughters for heroin money. The Hmong in Thailand now have a significant HIV problem (Vietnam is an unknown, as is China, where there are 5 million Hmong).

If it is true that suffering is a magnet for HIV, that it is drawn to add yet another burden to people who already have many, this latest twist in the fate of the Hmong only makes sense. HIV will further devastate an already ravaged people.

14. Other genders: *katoeys, waria, hinjras, toms* and *dees*

The great mother created three beings, the first man, the first woman, and the first *katoey*.

Lanna Thai Origin Story

Man or woman, boy or girl, male or female; straight, gay or bisexual – these categories of sex, gender, and sexual preference seem straightforward. They make biological sense. They come out of our world and have shaped it, from Adam and Eve to the nuclear family. What it means to be a man may vary across time, place and culture; what it means to be male we think of as much less varied – it's the birds and the bees . . . until you look at bees for a while, and realize that their genders are not so simple. Queens are made and not born (she who is fed royal jelly develops the great reproductive reservoir). Gender, for bees, is a task category, determined by the needs of the hive as much as by individual biology. Birds are not so straightforward, either. A subset of male ostriches prefers to live with other males, developing elaborate dances done with flexible necks and ticklish tails; some will kill any ostrich chicks they see. Herring gulls have high rates of female–female coupling. Lesbian gulls mate for life (does this sound familiar?) and lay double batch after double batch of unfertilized eggs.

What does it say of our clean dichotomies of sex that some cultures think there are three genders? Or that everyone is bisexual, or that no one is? Or that there are two kinds of women, one female and one male, but only one kind of male, who can have sex with both kinds of women and still be straight? Adam and Eve, and . . . Eve's half-sister? There are three genders in traditional Thai culture: men, women, and *katoey*, the last category being persons born with male bodies, who perceive themselves (and are perceived by others)

163

as female. They take on female dress, speak the female dialect, live from childhood through life as women, though of a special kind.

The origin story of the northern Thais serves as their version of *Genesis*.

The great mother created three beings, the first man, the first woman, and the first *katoey*. The *katoey* was jealous of first man's love for his wife, and killed her to have first man for his own. Because the *katoey* was also male, the marriage with first man was childless. The great mother killed them both and started again, creating second man, second woman, and second *katoey*. This time the second *katoey* felt his male energy, and was jealous of the man. He killed him, but wanted to live with the second woman as a sister, not a wife. Again the union was childless and again the great mother killed them both. When she created third man, third woman and third *katoey*, she pulled the third *katoey* aside and told him that he must let the man and woman live together and produce children so that creation could go on. The *katoey* would have a special role, but had to accept this marriage. The *katoey* agreed, and the Lanna people came into being, filling the valley with their offspring.

It is a strange story to western ears. The *katoey* is an ambiguous and potent figure, who must be compelled to make peace with both men and women so that the world can be populated. (S)he is something of a wild card, a dangerous element, but creation is not complete without her/him. Each time the genders are made anew, there are three.

When we started interviewing soldiers in the Thai army about sex with other men, we got a somewhat low response rate; 3.7% said they'd had sex with another man at least once in their lives. This seemed low, not only because Thais tend to be candid about sex, given the right interview environment, but because other groups had already reported rates as high as 14%, also among Thai soldiers. One of our interviewers, a young Thai man from Chiang Mai, and a native dialect speaker, suggested that our questions were the problem. We were asking, 'Have you ever had sex with another man?' using the Thai word *puchai*, man. Why should that be confusing? Because man does not include *katoey*. We then asked, 'Have you ever had sex with another man, or with a *katoey*?' The response rate more than doubled. The problem was that there really are three genders in northern Thai culture, and we had asked about only two of them.

What is a *katoey*? Biologically speaking, it is a normal male, as far as modern science goes. The word itself is thought to come from archaic Khmer: '*ka*' is derived from the word for person, '*toey*' from a word signifying 'other', or 'stranger', literally, another kind of person. Not far, perhaps, from the English 'queer'. Are *katoeys*, the often beautiful and always ultra-feminine Thai ladies (with penises and scrotums) born or made? Male or female? Gay or straight? My friend, the lovely Nadia from Pattaya, can answer all of these questions without skipping a beat. She was born the way she is. She is a *katoey*, which means being a special kind of woman, not a man. She has *jai ying*, a woman's heart. And she is 100% straight: gay men do not interest Nadia. Having an affair with another *katoey* would be either incest or lesbianism, and she is into neither. She wants a real man. And, in Thai culture at least, real men want her.

In the army data, several of the men who said they had had sex with *katoeys* did not have sex with anyone else, not other 'men' or other 'women', just *katoey*. A fourth gender? But most of the men who'd been with *katoeys* also reported many other partners: wives, girlfriends, female sex workers. In fact, these men (who we might be tempted to call 'bisexual', although they certainly wouldn't be) had, on average, more female partners than the men who had only female partners. When I pointed out this finding (it came from an analysis I was doing and I did not, at first, believe it, much less understand it) to a Thai colleague, he said 'Oh yes. They are just *nak tio*,' a rough translation of which would be 'hard-core party animals'. And they had the HIV rates to show it: 18% were infected by the age of 21, as opposed to 12% of men who had sex only with women.

Thai men like *katoey* for several reasons. In purely erotic terms, they will do things, like oral sex, that Thai women, especially social equals like wives, are taught to think of as dirty. They are described as 'tight' and 'dry,' references to the muscular anal sphincter. But like good Thai women, they will support a man, work to put food on his table, and tolerate infidelity with other women. One Thai friend told me that his mother was very upset when he had a young male lover – such boys cost money; they want nice clothes; they make demands. She was greatly relieved when he brought home a *katoey*, because, as she said, 'The *katoey* will take care of you, not the other way around' – Thai practicality at its best.

In traditional times the *katoey* had a lot of work to do to keep up feminine appearances: shaving; make-up; false breasts; concealing male genitalia, should a partner want this hidden. They did not, like the *hinjras* of India, self-castrate. Now, of course, there are female hormones; breast, lip and buttock implants; plastic surgery to reduce the ears or the nose; and, finally, castration and vaginoplasty: the surgical creation of female genitals out of male ones. This process – transsexual surgery, or gender 're-assignment' – is reserved for very particular cases in the West, cases of what we call true transsexualism. This is a relatively rare condition, characterized by lifelong, persistently held beliefs and feelings of having been born in the wrong body. In the US and Europe, surgeons will operate only after a person has had a minimum (in the US, two years) of psychological counseling to be sure that this is what they want. Often, two independent psychiatric evaluations are further required. This is to ensure that the gender-identity issue is the real one, and that there is not some other, underlying pathology which would drive a man to want to be castrated, or a woman to want to have bilateral mastectomies, a hysterectomy, and to go through puberty again.

In Thailand, all that is needed is the money. Transsexual surgery is done on demand, and many *katoey* have undertaken it. Are they the same as what we call 'transsexuals'? Or are they really a second form of woman choosing to become the first kind, the one without a penis? Nadia, who has had the surgery, is again clear on this issue, which I raised with her one drunken evening in Bangkok: she is still a *katoey*, but a more complete one.

Do these traditions survive, or did they ever exist, elsewhere? The Laos, being first cousins of the Thai, also have *katoey*. The identical term is used. Laotian attitudes appear to be similar to Thai ones, although the unanimous sentiment (in Vientiane and Luang Prabang) is that Thai *katoey* are more beautiful because they can afford hormones – Lao *katoey* still look more like men in skirts. (Nadia's mother is Lao; she loves her son like the good daughter she's become.)

Burma has another ancient and still vibrant tradition: the *nat pwe* performers. The 37 *nats* of Burmese tradition are semi-divine beings, usually humans who met terrible deaths in the historical past, worshipped through shamanic trance-like ceremonies. *Nat pwes* are the festivals held to honor these deities. The priests and priestesses of this unique Burmese cult 'marry' the *nats* they serve, with male priests becoming 'wives'. When this mystic marriage has occurred, the *nat* priest takes on female clothing, speech, and behavior, becoming, as it were, a kind of holy drag queen. Their fantastic costumes, elaborate face paint, and wild dancing style can only be described as high camp. While many *nat* priests and worshipers are not gay, the great *nat pwe* festivals serve as Burma's gay and transvestite gatherings. The largest one, at sacred Mount Popa, is said to attract 20,000 gay Burmese, and must be one of the world's singular parties. During the pro-democracy uprising of 1988, Burma's transvestites and gays had their own section marching through the streets of Rangoon. They were active participants in the struggle against the military, and there is video footage of their liberating parade past the waiting guns.

The *waria* of Indonesia are another transgender group in the region, one which serves an interesting role in Muslim-dominated Java. *Waria* is a combination of the word *wanita*, woman, and *pria*, man. Most are transvestites, not transsexuals, and nearly all are sex workers. There are thought to be about 5,000 in Jakarta alone. Their clientele are young Indonesian men and boys, who use the *waria* to experiment with sex. In this Muslim society young men traditionally cannot begin sexual life with women until marriage. The *waria* provide an outlet which serves the dual role of protecting unmarried girls from sexual pressures and allowing young men some sexual release. As in Thailand, the great majority of these young men are 'heterosexual' in orientation, even if their sexual lives begin with transvestite partners.

One HIV study has been done among the *waria*; more than 600 were interviewed and agreed to HIV testing. The average number of sex partners per week was 8; most clients wanted to anally penetrate the *waria*, to have oral sex, or to have 'simulated vaginal intercourse' between the thighs, the intracrural sex favored by the classical Greeks. In 1994, surprisingly, none of these 600 or so transvestites was HIV-infected, despite very high risks (nearly all reported regular receptive anal sex without condoms). HIV rates in their young and sexually inexperienced partners are likely to be low, but the potential for rapid spread is real.

Malaysia also has its transvestites, as does Cambodia, the birthplace of the term *katoey*. India, a root civilization for all the cultures discussed, has her traditional transgender class, though the Indian tradition is something of a special case. There is an excellent discussion of this tradition in the *Kama Sutra*, the Sanskrit classic on sex and sexuality, which describes not only the third gender, but the kinds of intercourse men might have with them (in addition to what must surely be one of the world's earliest treatises on fellatio).

Indian civilization has an awesome ability to see almost anything in terms of the spirit. Prostitution still has a religious gloss in the hereditary temple prostitutes of Rajasthan. Poverty and nakedness, a life of ashes, are the revered garb of the Saddhu. And the Indian 'third gender', the *hinjra*, are called into service by the Divine Mother to serve her cult. There are very few ways permanently to 'lose' caste in India: you can get leprosy, a potent social leveler; you can become enlightened in this lifetime, triumphing over all karma, including a low birth; or you can become a *hinjra*. Unlike Thailand or Laos, where men who choose (or are born to) this path can stay with their families, in their communities, and live as ordinary women, the Indian *hinjra* becomes an instant outcast, leaving family, community, and caste. She usually joins a band of others like her, and takes up a life of wandering, street performing, begging, and prostitution, if she survives the initiation; many do not.

The initiation into the service of the Goddess is a sacrifice, offered with one swift slice of a knife – penis, scrotum, testicles. Those who survive have typically only a small scarred opening through which to urinate. Infections are common, as are strictures and chronic pain. To serve the Goddess fully, the initiate also plucks (not shaves – too easy!) all of the male body hair. There is one last step in this process: anal dilatation, usually using a wooden dildo set in a special chair, to prepare for a life of selling sex to straight men. (What we do for love!) Thai *katoeys* cross the educational and class spectrum, and are very much aware of HIV and STDs. By 1995, over 40% of rural *hinjra* had already acquired HIV. The virus is likely to wipe them out.

And the ladies? *Tom* is a Thai word adapted from 'tomboy', an Americanism for a girl with boyish behavior. *Dee*, another Thai expression, is a shortened form of the English 'lady'. *Tom* and *dee* have fairly precise equivalents in English: butch and femme, top and bottom, bulldyke and lipstick lesbian. It is immediately obvious that while words like *katoey* and *hinjra* are ancient, the words used to identify lesbians in Thai culture are very new and very much borrowed from other tongues and topographies. There is an old expression in Thai for sex between women: *lin phuen*, to 'play with friends', but this specifies an act, not a gender or type of woman; both words in this expression are gender-neutral. There may be an unwritten history of lesbian or female transgender traditions in Southeast Asia, but there is very little documentation available. Women's sexuality is (as always) much less discussed, studied and understood. The traditional 'third genders' are all variations on maleness approaching the female, not the other way around. Seen this way, the *katoey*, the *waria*, the *hinjra* are all forms of Asian male identity: they reflect, perhaps, much more how the societies they come from configure male gender and sexuality, not female. Women, even if men attempt to become them through radical self-mutiliation, remain hidden.

One does, however, see the occasional Thai woman in a suit and tie, with a brush cut, speaking the male dialect. If Thai society does not have a name for her, equivalent to *katoey*, she is still fully taking on a male role; such women are not rare, and they seem, in tolerant Thailand, at least, socially acceptable. I met one such person in Laos as well, in the entourage of the Minister of Forestry; we chatted for several minutes in Thai before I realized that the young bureaucrat was a woman. His voice, clothes, and hair were perfect, but you can't fake an adam's apple.

15. *Chaai chuay chaai*: men helping men

The box arrived one day at my office in Chiang Mai, brimming over with sheets of yellowing paper. It had come from Dr Chawalit's office, from a nurse named Khun Piyada, and it contained the results of five years' work with men and boys working in Chiang Mai's gay bars and clubs. It took some time to sort through the data, get it into shape for analysis, put it together, and understand what it all meant. Buried in these data was epidemiologic gold – a tremendous amount of information on bar-boys and their extraordinary risk of HIV infection, but also evidence that some men had been able to avoid the virus, despite years of selling sex.

Male commercial sex in Thailand is a very different affair from the heterosexual commercial scene. It is a much smaller branch of the industry, localized to essentially five sites: the cities of Bangkok and Chiang Mai, and the beach resorts of Pattaya, Phuket, and Hat Yai. The workers are not trafficked and not, by and large, debt-bonded. The sex is considerably more expensive, the pay better for workers. Even in the flesh trade, it's a man's world.

Most male sex workers in Thailand are heterosexual outside their work in bars; perhaps 60% say they prefer sex with women; about 15% are married. This information was in the box from Khun Piyada, and other groups had confirmed similar rates of heterosexual orientation among male prostitutes in Bangkok. This finding raises the important issue of 'bridge' populations; straight male sex workers may be an important link in chains of transmission between Thai women and Western gay men, groups that might otherwise interact little. The bridge goes both ways, of course: the Thai subtype E virus, so common among Thai heterosexuals, could also track from male sex workers to gay clients from all over the world. If this virus really is more infectious through sex than the subtype B virus found in most infected Western gay men, a new epidemic might be expected.

Sex work for men tends to be much shorter-term than it is for women. The average time in the business is six months, and about one-third of workers do it for two months or less. Women work an average of two years or more, and debt-bonded women often have to work this long before they begin to see any money. Men and boys, in contrast, sell sex for short-term financial needs, for fast cash. Most are rural men coming to the city for the first time; sex work is a starter's job, and it pays considerably better than menial labor or restaurant work, other typical first-time employments.

The clients are also a different group. Most Thai men cannot afford the drinks in a gay bar, much less one of the boys. The clients in the gay scene are well-heeled, and the workers report that about half their clients are not Thai, a much higher percentage than in the heterosexual market. Other Asians are represented, as are Europeans, Australians, and North Americans. In Hat Yai, on the Thai–Malaysian border, a significant part of the business is Malaysian men. A small minority of clients are women, or heterosexual couples. A small scene has been described on the island of Phuket, where Thai men specialize in providing sex (and entertainment) to Japanese women. Denied casual sex in their own country, a new generation of Japanese women look for it elsewhere.

Thai commercial gay bars are bizarre places, quite unlike what most gay men would recognize as a gay bar in the West: anywhere from ten to forty men hanging around in jock straps, with numbers pinned to their crotches; go-go boys dancing nude, or nearly so; live sex shows; 'captains' circulating, asking if any number strikes your fancy. These are not brothels – the sex happens elsewhere – making the gay bars rough equivalents of 'indirect' or higher-class straight establishments. Customers have to pay the bar to take a worker home; this is the source of the bar's income, along with drinks and cover charges for shows. What the sex worker gets is between him and the customer. Some bars specialize in offering weight lifters or boxer types; others have poetically beautiful young men in Tuxedos, or dressed up in traditional Thai formal wear, barefoot and bowing. *Katoeys* are rare in the commercial scene, except as drag-show performers. What clients want is muscular, clean-cut, athletic types – straight farm boys – which is, in fact, mostly what they get.

In the five years' work done by Khun Piyada, we found that, despite the short-term nature of their work, and much higher levels of empowerment and education, male sex workers were none the less getting infected with HIV at high, steady rates. These men had, in fact, the highest rates of new HIV infection of any group of men in Asia; from 1989 to 1995 a regular 12% per year were getting HIV. This was in addition to the 20% of men who were already positive on any cross-sectional look, making gay-bar work about as deadly an occupation as one can imagine. This was hard to reconcile with what seemed to be much better working conditions than those found among female sex workers. These were Thai men, not tribal boys; many were literate; some were university students making pocket money while they studied. Two other findings helped to clarify the situation. Men who had worked longer in the business should have had higher rates, since they would have had many more opportunities for infection. They did not; their rates were lower, and fell progressively over time. This suggested that if men had time to learn about safer sex, they did better at staying uninfected. The second finding was more straightforward: men who said they 'sometimes', 'most often', or 'almost always' used condoms had the same high rate as men who said they 'rarely' or 'never' used them. Only men who said they 'always' used condoms for anal sex were protected. Not a surprise. What was surprising was that condom use was not universal; it was lower than among men in the Thai army: only 56% of male sex workers said they 'always' used condoms. Even in the cheapest brothels, female sex workers were doing better. During the five years of the study, the nurses from the ministry had been giving out free condoms to all the workers, the bars all had them prominently displayed, sex workers asked to show condoms nearly always had some on hand. What was wrong?

The problem was, and is, a complex one, and it is far from solved. The Ministry of Health program was only able to visit each bar twice a year, so many short-term workers missed it entirely. The data suggested that men new to the business were the least skilled at using condoms, and at avoiding HIV. Sexual orientation did not seem to matter. Men who said they were 'men', 'gay kings', 'gay queens', or 'katoey' all had roughly the same risk. The crucial time for HIV risk appeared to be the learning phase of sex work, the first few weeks or months on the job, before workers knew how to insist on condom use, and before they themselves were skilled in safe anal sex practices. Most reported that foreign clients were easier to negotiate condom use with than their own countrymen. Thai clients more often demanded anal intercourse and did not want to wear condoms. How to intervene?

With several friends, we developed the concept of a sex workers' group, which would train men working in the industry to be peer educators. This network would identify any new workers in the bars, and get to them with frank practical advice on avoiding HIV before they became infected. We called the group *Chaai Chuay Chaai* – men helping men. (To 'help', *chuay*, is a Thai euphemism for masturbation, so the name has a second meaning, immediately clear to Thais.) The group got funding from the Australian government, and we were in business. We had five volunteers, all sex workers or ex-sex workers, who regularly visited all the gay bars that would have them, the cruising areas, and the street hustler scenes of nighttown Chiang Mai – places they had all worked and knew intimately. They came back from their shifts with some incredible tales to tell.

One bar did have some trafficked workers. These were Shan and Burmese who had been brought to Thailand on construction crews. When their road work or construction jobs ended, some of the younger and more handsome ones had been recruited into sex work. Several workers turned out to be SLORC soldiers who had defected from the army, snuck into Thailand, and ended up in the bars as illegal aliens. There were boys from Laos. There was much more drug abuse than the boys had reported to the visiting nurse teams; glue- and thinner-sniffing was common, as was ecstasy, amphetamines, and heavy alcohol use. And there *were* some real brothels. These were very clandestine, strictly Thai establishments without the usual bars or restaurant businesses as covers. Three were found. These places were all private homes, open in the afternoon, when the workers got out of school. Local men came for cheap sex with schoolboys, virtually all of whom were supporting drug habits by selling sex. Reaching them was dangerous, and had to be done with caution. There was also a small pedophile scene, operating out of several bars, where men could arrange for sex with boys as young as 8 or 9. As soon as the volunteers reached these places, the children promptly disappeared; these kids proved almost impossible to track down. We started working with a local group that tried to offer housing and support to homeless street kids, and found that many had been part of this pedophile scene; more than half had HIV infection in 1995.

Our volunteers were giving out a lot of condoms and lubricants, and counseling all over the city, night after night. After a year, we eagerly awaited the results from the ministry survey of the bars. Were we having an effect? No, we weren't. HIV rates were steady, despite continuing efforts on the part of the Ministry, despite *Chaai Chuay Chaai*, despite the national education campaign which seemed to be working with so many other groups. Gay commercial sex was not getting any safer, and that is where the situation stands.

Several other countries in the region have male commercial sex scenes in addition to Thailand: Sri Lanka and the Philippines are the most commonly cited. Indonesia has a local trade in transvestites; Bali is known for a significant sex tourist scene with gay bars and beach boys, and for an international clientele. What makes Thailand somewhat different is that it is easily the most tolerant and open country in Asia for gay men, for commercial sex patrons, but also for gay men who are not interested in commercial sex. For this group, Bangkok is the new Amsterdam, the New York or Paris of the region. When you go out to the non-commercial bars and clubs of gay Bangkok, you meet Singaporeans, Malaysians, Indonesians, Taiwanese, Indians, Koreans, Japanese, Filipinos, Laotians – men reveling in the freedom of big, hot discos, fabulously louche gay saunas, disinterested police.

There is nothing else quite like this in Asia. There is one gay disco in Vientiane, although it is quite underground, and caters to an almost entirely Lao crowd. The place was absolutely packed when I found it – with the help of a sweet, emaciated Lao transvestite – a roomy dance-hall full of young Laos dancing to the latest house music. The police arrived promptly at midnight, turned on the lights, and emptied the place with dispatch. Kuala Lumpur has a gay scene, but it is limited to two bars, and one small district. KL gays love to party in Bangkok, free of the threat of closure, police raids, and exposure. Consensual sex between adult men is a felony in Singapore, and, like most 'crimes' in the rich city-state, it is prosecuted to the full extent of the law. Singapore canes and imprisons homosexuals; anal intercourse can get you five years. So Singapore's gays too, can be found getting down in Bangkok (caning is available, but only on request).

16. Prisons and prisoners

Owing to drug abuse, there is also a high prevalence of HIV/AIDS in prisons. Prisoners are always afraid to get injections in the jail hospital because of AIDS. When administering injections, the doctors give only half or less than half of the phial to one patient, giving the rest to another patient from the same needle and syringe, this almost guaranteeing that any blood-carried infections will spread. This means that the doctors can get away with using less medicines per patient.

The following are the usual implements used for beating prisoners:

1. Leather-coated pipe
2. Wooden stick
3. Stick made from three interlaced pieces of cane
4. Solid bamboo stick about 3–4 ft in length
5. Hard plastic water pipe

Cries from Insein: a Report on Conditions for Political Prisoners in Burma. (ABSDF, 1996)

On 2 August 1996, a man died in Yangon General Hospital, having been brought there, near death, from Insein Prison in Burma. His name was U Hla Than. He was an elected member of the Burmese Parliament, the body which won the 1990 elections but was never allowed to convene. He was 52 years old. Opposition groups immediately claimed that he had been tortured to death, a common enough occurence in Insein Prison, which Amnesty International has repeatedly cited for its gross violations of human rights and for the use of torture. The military dictatorship, SLORC, claimed he died of tuberculosis. Aung San Suu Kyi (who has just been put under *de facto* house arrest again) made a public statement in October about the death of her colleague which contrasted with both of these positions. The MP had been tortured, and he had died of tuberculosis, but neither of these facts were sufficient to tell the whole truth. His tuberculosis was a complication of AIDS, Aung San Suu Kyi wanted to stress. His HIV infection was a complication of his imprisonment, and his imprisonment was for the crime of having been democratically elected. He was not known to be a heroin user or to have been involved in homosexual activities while in prison – as an older man and a political prisoner famous among his people, he was somewhat spared from these threats. But like so many prisoners in Burma's jails, he had been offered food (a single hard-boiled egg is standard, according to survivors) in exchange for blood. Blood-collection equipment in Burma's gulag is routinely re-used without sterilization, as documented above in the account of Win Naing Oo, a young man incarcerated for three years in Insein Prison for participating in the 1988 student movement against the junta. In U Hla Than, another Burmese democracy leader was martyred, the instrument being not a 'hard plastic water pipe' or a bullet, but the human immunodeficiency virus.

Burma has been called a prison with 43 million inmates. There is some truth in this, certainly if we consider the human-rights situation, and the severe restrictions on Burmese citizens' freedom of speech, assembly, and travel. The situation of the prisons within this prison-state are an extremity within an extremity. Heroin is available, for a price, as are raw opium, concentrated opium oil, marijuana, and valium. Homosexual rape of younger prisoners is common: they are selected on arrival by senior prisoners and the leaders of criminal networks within the jails. Condoms are not available.

Nor are condoms provided to prisoners in the Thai, the Malaysian, the Indian, or, for the most part, the US prison systems. A senior Thai prosecutor told me that almost any sentence longer than three years was considered tantamount to a death sentence in the prison in Chiang Mai, since prisoners held any longer than this were dying 'like flies' of AIDS. It is a terrible irony of the Thai epidemic that a 1988 national amnesty offered to prisoners (owing to an important anniversary) first released an unknown number of HIV-infected men into the country. Needle sharing and unprotected homosexual sex had spread HIV extensively among these men. Within months of their release, the Thai epidemic was under way.

HIV prevention in prisons has been an abysmal, even criminal failure worldwide. In Asia it has been no better handled than in most prison systems. What makes the Burmese and Thai situations so lethal is that HIV rates are already high enough among young men, such that prison acts as an accelerator. Indeed, among addicts in Thailand, having been incarcerated is the single most important difference between men who have HIV and those who do not. HIV infection in Thai addicts is highly correlated with having been jailed.

The United States of America, to its lasting shame as a nation born to embody freedom, has the highest incarceration rate in the world: approximately 2.6% of all Americans over 18 in 1993, almost 5 million people. South Africa used to be a close second, but has since dropped out of the running, leaving us essentially alone among developed nations in our fervor to imprison our citizens. As befits the new era of privatization, prisons are now profit-making enterprises, with privately operated prisons picking up the slack of the overwhelmed public system. In a stunning ironic twist worthy of Gogol, prisons now mean jobs. One phrase (is it actually true?) has been repeated till it has lost the power to shock: 'There are more young black men in prison than in college in America today.' If we cannot prevent this generation of young people from contracting HIV while in custody, because of squeamishness over their having sex in jail and our denial of the availability of drugs, 'death row' will have a whole new meaning, similar to what it now means to go to jail in Thailand or Burma. While we deny incarcerated persons condoms, interviews with ex-inmates in New York prisons suggest that they are all too aware of the risks; inmates use rubber gloves, even used plastic wrap from prison kitchens, in an attempt to protect themselves from HIV.

No one deserves such treatment, not first time non-violent offenders caught on the wrong side of the 'war on drugs', and not repeat offenders. If the law finds that a person should be punished with death, so be it, but we should do this honestly, not pretend that we are not doing so. A death sentence, it could be argued, is what the denial of regular supplies of condoms amounts to.

17. The media

Freedom of the press is rare in Southeast Asia. Of the seven countries discussed here, only Thailand and Cambodia (for now) have vigorous print media which openly criticize government bodies and political figures. There are two English-language dailies in the Thai Kingdom: the *Bangkok Post*, and *The Nation*, both of which cover local and international news with thorough rigor. Both have also covered the HIV/AIDS crisis unflinchingly, and with considerably less sensationalism than the Thai-language papers (the most popular of which are roughly equivalent to the US or British tabloids, with the same emphasis on violence, 'human interest' stories, and local crime). *The Nation* is very much the 'newspaper of record' on Burma; its journalists have extensive contacts with the Burmese opposition, which give them access to stories and events not covered elsewhere. These Thai dailies have a wide impact; they are often the only printed news available in Thailand's neighbors. The *Bangkok Post* can be bought discreetly from street vendors in Ho Chi Minh City and Vientiane, a godsend when you can get it. After a stint in Rangoon, Beijing, or Laos, where print, television and radio are all government-controlled and heavily censored, it's ever a pleasure to be back in Thailand, to have access to information. You feel that you're at last being treated like an adult again, not a child that military censors have to protect and control.

The *New Light of Myanmar*, SLORC's house organ and the only English-language newspaper in Burma, is arguably the worst in a bad lot. A typical headline reads 'Entrepreneurs of Upper Myanmar demand internal, external destructionist groups stop making fabrications, machinations', a convoluted way of saying SLORC is furious with the elected leadership for calling for economic sanctions against them. The paper includes, every day, a boxed section called 'People's Desire', which could have been written by Madame Mao in her Cultural Revolution heyday:

- Oppose those relying on external elements, acting as stooges, holding negative views.
- Oppose those trying to jeopardize stability of the State and progress of the nation.
- Oppose foreign nations interfering in internal affairs of the State.
- Crush all internal and external destructive elements as the common enemy.

In the context of Burma, the 'crush' in the last bullet is an unveiled threat, its meaning not lost on citizens. It used to be said that in the old Soviet Union it was easy to know the truth: whoever *Pravda* was denouncing was good; whoever was being called a hero was a villain; what was denied was probably true; what was trumpeted as truth could only be lie. This same inversion applies to SLORC's 'People's Desire'. The people of Burma have expressed their desire, through free elections, and the military was routed. The people, their chosen leaders, and the international community, know only too well that SLORC are the real 'destructive internal elements'. With heroin exports doubling during their eight years in power (according to a 1996 US State Department report, based on satellite imaging of poppy cultivation acreage), and domestic use soaring even faster, who else is 'threatening the stability of the nation'? (*Wall Street Journal* editorial, 18 November 1996, 'The Bad Neighbor'.)

The *New Light of Myanmar* has been pushing the line that the HIV epidemic in Burma is slowing down. Doctors and nurses have risked their lives to tell journalists and researchers that this is not so, and that they have been warned to stop reporting new cases, at least since 1994. The crude propaganda fools no one, but the lack of real information endangers all. The same holds true for the country's only television station, Myanmar Television. If any senior SLORC general is unfamiliar, just switch on the evening news: you will see them all in turn, kissing babies, offering food to monks, visiting factories. The monotony of the images on totalitarian television is startling. No one smiles when the TV cameras pan the generals' audiences; no one moves. At their parades, there are no crowds, no traffic. Reality is orchestrated to the last detail. But the result is laughably far from convincing; this is one reason why the odd statement by a businessman or diplomat passing through Rangoon that things are improving in Myanmar always rings disingenuous; switch on the evening news and you'd have to be blind and deaf not to see how crude and controlling this regime is, how afraid of information. This makes the journalists who cover Burma a special breed, and the information they get out precious. The tragedy is that accurate information is even harder to disseminate inside Burma; this holds true for China, Laos, and Vietnam as well. The implications for public health cannot be underestimated. To be effective, public health has to be a partnership between trusted public sectors and an informed public. The public's right to know and its right to choose are essential elements of effective intervention. If the media are seen as serving only government organs, how can a mistrustful public be expected to respond to AIDS messages? It could be posited that a free and vigorous flow of information is a key component of any country's ability to cope with threats to public health and well-being. The difference between the Thai and Burmese press is yet another indicator of Thailand's hopeful HIV prognosis and Burma's despairing one.

All the more reason, then, to question the quality of HIV/AIDS reporting in the media. If you are active in a research-based field, attend conferences, and keep up to date with the literature of your discipline, you may often find that the relationship between what is new and important in your field and what becomes news in wider media can be arbitrary, even capricious. Scientific misconduct, alleged or proven, is often big news. The battle between the French and American teams over who first isolated the HIV is an example: the controversy was headline news for several years after most HIV researchers had moved on to other issues. Nevertheless, the relationship between the professional literature and the lay media is an important one; most people get their information from the lay news, not from peer-reviewed journals, and, in the case of public health, the general public is a key target audience for new information. The interests and needs of the lay media, however, can be strikingly different from that of the professions.

This is the situation that prevailed at Berlin in 1993, at the ninth International Conference on AIDS. The hottest news story to come out of the conference was 'AIDS Without HIV', the finding that a very small number of persons had been found with illnesses that looked like AIDS, but who appeared not to be HIV-infected. This was picked up by the wire services, the television networks, CNN and the BBC, and all the major American and European print media. It was a new 'hook' for AIDS stories, a new angle. Dr Anthony Fauci, Director of the US National Institutes of Allergy and Infectious Diseases (NIAID) was all over the television during the conference, and held a packed press conference on his return to the US pledging that NIAID would immediately put the full weight of its resources into investigating the seven American cases of what the media had dubbed 'HIV-negative AIDS'. And NIAID did spend some US$10 million investigating these cases. They turned out to be what virtually all the scientists present (including Dr Fauci) knew they were as soon as the cases were first described: a grab-bag of unrelated illnesses and immune disorders, including several mis-diagnosed cancers and a familial immune disorder in a mother and daughter. Immune deficiency disorders are not new; they predate AIDS, and there will be sporadic cases long after HIV is defeated, should it ever be. All of the immunologists present knew this, and many, like Dr Fauci, had built their careers studying these diseases before 1981, when the new immune disorder, then called GRID (for gay-related immune deficiency) and now AIDS, was first described.

There was a vastly more important story that broke at Berlin, over the same days as 'HIV-negative AIDS', which had a very different fate. This was the first presentation of national data on HIV from India, a country which had previously reported little information on the epidemic. When I saw the presentation of this information, in a huge half-empty hall at the Congress, I wept from about the third slide to the last. India was just starting surveillance, and had not begun anything like a national prevention program, but the virus was years ahead of the authorities; the numbers were unparalleled – and they have been borne out – unlike the red herring that caused the media frenzy. India now has the worst HIV problem in the world, forcing the World Health Organization to sharply increase its forecasts of the global epidemic to accommodate India's vast at-risk population. In Berlin the estimate was that at least 1 million Indians were infected; the estimate is now closer to 5 million, and rising.

The news from India was not important as far as the international media were concerned. It was more of the same, not a new hook, and it was almost universally ignored. For those of us working in the field, however, this was the bombshell of the meeting, which would require a change in thinking, in priorities, in strategy. This split, between what gets covered and what scientists and researchers actually worry about, has been one of the painful realities of this politically and socially contentious epidemic. It was made all the more disturbing by the position subsequently taken by the Indian authorities: the Indian Minister of Health, speaking a year later at an Asian forum on AIDS, insisted that India would be protected by 'traditional Indian family values', and did not need to deal with condoms, or sex education, or sexually transmitted diseases.

What are the responsibilities of the media? How has coverage affected the crisis? The 'HIV-negative AIDS' fiasco cost the US taxpayers some millions of dollars to investigate, but this may have been less important than several other outcomes. There has long been a small minority of scientists and activists who have maintained, despite a rising mountain of evidence, that HIV is not the cause of AIDS, or not the only sufficient cause. Their campaign was certainly aided, for a time, by the story. There is an even smaller but quite vocal minority, who insist that the AIDS epidemic is itself a fiction, a conspiracy, or that its numbers are hugely overblown. There are several different streams of thought at work here: new-age environmentalists who feel that 'the planet' has AIDS, that dolphins are dying of immune deficiency, and that it is the destruction of the environment that is causing similar immune problems in humans; gay activists who feel that the epidemic is a conspiracy to limit their sexual freedom; another minority which believes that the gravity of AIDS has been vastly overestimated in an attempt to increase research moneys. For many of these groups, finding 'AIDS without HIV' was proof positive for their theories, a vindication of sorts. There was no shortage of such persons willing to be interviewed by the media. After all the losses, the deaths of patients, friends, lovers, and colleagues, I equate the statement that 'the AIDS epidemic does not exist' as roughly equivalent to the revisionist historical position that the holocaust didn't happen. It is the gravest possible insult to the fallen, and a dangerous and real threat to those alive.

What about crimes of omission? Would the Indian Minister of Health have been so complacent if the international media had picked up the story of India's catastrophe? If CNN had gone to the tiger-cage brothels of Bombay after the conference, or sent correspondents to one of the thousands of private, unregulated blood banks that dot Indian cities? This is the other side of poor reporting: the neglect of failures in public policy. Because the media have the power to focus attention, to put pressure on leaders and decision makers, to educate and to alert, its failure to do so is all the more disturbing.

The responsibility, however, is not the media's alone. Scientists and public health officials have often done poorly in educating and cultivating journalists, in being transparent and accessible, and in sharing information. Good journalists have to be open to information from any and all sources. It is their professional responsibility to assess the veracity of the information they receive, to check sources and verify reports. But public health officials and the wider scientific establishment are not always eager to speak to journalists. Science compels us first of all to discuss only what we have evidence for, tentative and uncertain findings are not for public consumption, limiting our ability to speak frankly when a story is breaking. Then there is the problem of the ownership of information. All the *New York Times* stories in the world are worth less to a practicing scientist than one lead paper in the *New England Journal of Medicine*. Since scientific publications are generally peer-reviewed, and the review and rewriting process nearly always takes several months, researchers have to withhold information and findings that are under review. By the time the findings appear in the scientific literature, public interest may have moved on. This was very much the case with 'HIV-negative AIDS'. An exhaustive investigation into the cases was published several months after the Berlin meeting in the *New England Journal of Medicine* by the US Centers for Disease Control. By then, the media were less interested, and the scientific community already knew the outcome of the story. The publication was a non-event.

A more recent interaction of the American media with the Thai AIDS epidemic was the result of a publication in the journal *Science* of a finding by a Harvard–Chiang Mai University collaborative group that the subtype E HIV appeared to grow more efficiently in cell cultures from the genital tract than in lymphocytes, the white blood cells of the blood and lymphatic tissues. This finding suggested that subtype E might be 'tropic,' or preferentially infect genital tissues over blood. The researchers postulated that this might be the underlying cause of the heterosexual epidemic in Thailand (and in Asia in general), where transmission from male to female and from female to male through vaginal intercourse appeared to be more efficient than such spread in the US, the difference being that while spread through needle sharing (blood) and anal intercourse ('bloodier' than vaginal sex) still seemed to account for the majority of American infections with subtype B, a blood-tropic virus, heterosexual sex was the predominant means of spread with subtype E. This was picked up by television journalists as the possibility of a 'super-virus', a mutant strain that was more infectious, more deadly, and more likely to affect heterosexuals than homosexuals. Phone calls, faxes, and e-mails flew between Chiang Mai and New York; a television news crew from a major network appeared soon after in Thailand, a camera crew showed up at Johns Hopkins. It was a hot story. But there were major problems. The 'super-virus' concept was supported by very little evidence. The Harvard–Chiang Mai University re-searchers who proposed it were suggesting that much more work needed to be done before it even be called a theory. The study had shown a difference in *culture* characteristics, meaning differences in the 'test tube', not in human beings. And HIV notoriously behaves very differently inside and outside the body; past experiences have made researchers cautious in generalizing laboratory findings to patients, much less to countries, or, in this case, continents. Perhaps more importantly, the news coverage failed to mention the most important finding to come out of the Thai epidemic – one that *had* been proven in humans beings – that high rates of condom use had dramatically reduced new rates of HIV in Thailand. However potent the subtype E virus was, however more likely to spread between men and women during sex, condoms were just as effective in preventing it as they had been shown to be in preventing spread of subtype B between men. The journalists who spoke to me about the 'super-virus' theory all wanted doom and gloom on the Thai epidemic. (For doom and gloom, I suggested, they could send a crew to Burma or Cambodia. None did.) I could interest none in Thailand's successes. They were seeking to cover something like killer bees, or the Ebola outbreak in Zaire; they wanted a sensationally bad story that would click with American viewers, not moderate hope that prevention campaigns might save millions of lives in far-away parts of the world. Or at home.

I was on a flight from Washington to Bangkok about a week after the media blitz over the 'super virus'. The man sitting next to me was an American of Thai background, on his way to a family reunion. We chatted for a while, and he asked me about my work. When I said I worked with HIV in Thailand he visibly jumped in his seat. 'Holy shit, you work with that stuff? That's the worst bug in the world. It might spread through the air. I just saw a show about it on TV. My wife wanted me to cancel my trip.'

18. Activists

Humanity's innate desire is for freedom, truth, and democracy. The non-violent 'people power' movements that have arisen in various parts of the world in recent years have indisputably shown that human beings can neither tolerate nor function properly under tyrannical conditions.

Tenzin Gyatso, His Holiness the Fourteenth Dalai Lama of Tibet

Demands for prevention rarely get protestors out on the streets. Vaccines have had few vocal advocates since the polio scares of the 1930s and 1940s, except those demanding compensation for putatively vaccine-related damage to their children. Demands for care, for access to treatment, have created mass movements, for no disease perhaps more spectacularly than for AIDS. AIDS activism brought about changes in the price of drugs (AZT, after activists chained themselves to the doors of the New York Stock Exchange, delaying the opening of the world's largest financial market), altered the way the US Food and Drug Administration approves new agents (after a series of actions there), and forced the Centers for Disease Control to review the very definition of the disease (after ACT-UP occupied the roof of their Atlanta office building). While not all the outcomes of AIDS activism have been beneficial to people with the disease, or to researchers, the cumulative effect of public pressure can be seen in the astonishingly wide array of new treatments now under evaluation or recently approved, in the anti-viral combination therapies, and in the huge research investments that have tested their clinical efficacy. For people with HIV/AIDS in the West, 1995–96 was a watershed; there are, at last, anti-retroviral therapies with specific activity against HIV. We now have the technology (quantitative viral load testing) to measure viral responsiveness to these drugs in patients taking them, allowing for rational and informed decisions about when to change agents, when to stop them altogether, when to initiate them in a person seemingly well but in whom the virus has begun aggressive replication. I have seen friends who were at death's door begin to gain weight, grow back their hair, get off disability and go back to work within three to six months after starting on the new three-drug regimes. This kind of progress would not have occurred without the immense resources appropriated to the NIH (specifically NIAID) under the Bush and Clinton administrations. But those resources might never have been mustered had it not been for the committed and effective activists on the front lines of confrontation. Who will ever forget ACT-UP's infiltration of the evening news in New York, at the height of the Gulf War, shouting 'Fight AIDS, not Arabs' to a stunned anchorman?

Sadly, these potent drugs and the measures of their utility are even more expensive than the older agents (AZT, ddI, ddC) and even less likely to be available to the great majority of people with AIDS worldwide. In countries where people die for lack of cheap generic drugs like penicillin or quinine, they are as likely to be available as coronary bypass surgery. An elite handful, who usually seek medical care in places like Singapore or Switzerland, will get them, but few others. Only HIV prevention is going to save appreciable numbers of lives, but where is the activist constituency for condoms?

Thailand has had one activist, Khun Meechai Viravaidya, a prominent citizen who made condom promotion a personal crusade. Khun Meechai used a promotion tactic all too often ignored by Western activists: humor. He appealed to the Thai sense of *sanuk* -- fun -- using condom flowers, giving condom bouquets to ladies, spreading a message that stressed the 'sex-positive', and the maintenance of pleasure that safer sex could mean in the era of AIDS. Wherever and whenever he appeared, at society balls or at public schools, he gave out condoms. He started a chain of restaurants, called 'Cabbages and Condoms', where all diners received condoms with their meals. So associated did he become with condom use that the slang word for condom in central Thai became 'a Meechai', and using a *meechai* became synonymous with practicing safer sex. As a member of the Thai elite, Khun Meechai had considerable access to the media and to Thai decision makers, access that he used to promote condoms tirelessly, but always with wit, humor, and appeals to the Thai sense of tolerance and sexual pleasure. While direct effects are always difficult to measure, there is no question that his early and energetic efforts contributed to the rapid nationwide increase in condom use that makes Thailand unique, at least for now, in Asia. In a promising sign that his message may have a regional impact as well, Khun Meechai received Asia's highest humanitarian award, the Magsaysay Prize, last year.

So far, however, Thailand is unique in having produced a Khun Meechai. The other ASEAN states trail, particularly as regards grass-roots activism. The long incubation period of HIV is again a factor here. By the time friends, lovers, spouses and children are sick and dying from AIDS, and given the time it always seems to take before such people and communities organize and try to take action, the time for early prevention is usually past. This is certainly the scenario in rural Thailand, and in Malaysia and Cambodia, the three countries in the region that, so far, have appreciable activist movements.

Northern Thailand now has more than 60 self-help groups for people with HIV/AIDS. Most have come together seeking treatments, including the largest, *Pheun Cheewit*, New Life Friends, which has over 5,000 members in the Chiang Mai valley. New Life Friends was actually an unwitting creation of the Thai Ministry of Health. In 1994, a herbalist in northern Thailand was making a name selling a herbal remedy for HIV which, he claimed, could make people go from being HIV-positive to HIV-negative. People flocked to him. The great majority, of course, were getting no other treatment, and were never going to afford AZT, the only AIDS drug then available in Thailand. The Ministry was rightly concerned that the man was a profiteer, exploiting people with AIDS for money, of which he was reportedly making plenty. The herbalist was shut down, causing instant uproar among the hundreds of people to whom he had offered, if nothing else, hope. Galvanized, they formed New Life Friends to lobby the government for access to the banned herbal treatment. In classic Thai fashion, a deal was struck: New Life Friends would be recognized as a 'club', members would pay a small monthly fee of 50 Baht (about US$2, well within most Thai pocketbooks) and would then have access to the herbal therapy, which would be free to club members. The club quickly caught on, and now serves not only as a mechanism for access to care, but as a social group, a community center, and a place to look for work.

Two other strands of activism have emerged in the Thai epidemic, from two very different groups in society: sex workers and their advocates; and the *sangha*, the monastic community.

Early on in the Thai epidemic there was tremendous fear of people with AIDS. Fear of contagion born of misunderstandings that were only natural given the lack of general awareness at the community level, the newness of the disease and its high lethality. Finding places to get care was a real problem; many clinics and hospitals turned the early cases away. Finding places to live, and then to die, became even more problematic. The long-term solution was clearly going to have to be home care; this the authorities recognized and promoted, as did the very active Thai Red Cross, which soon began support programs, and has now trained thousands of home-care givers. But in the short term there was a real crisis: people with AIDS were living in parks, isolated like lepers at the outskirts of villages, abandoned by families to the street. The Thai *wat*, the Buddhist temple, has always been a place of refuge. Children without care-givers have long been 'given' to *wats*; widows and childless elderly are often found staying at them, as are young people between jobs, even criminals hiding from the law, or AWOL soldiers.

The first Thai *wat* to offer refuge, and to create an AIDS hospice for the dying, was in Lopburi, in the lower north. The Abbot, a progressive and powerful figure in Thai monasticism, faced considerable criticism for opening his center. (He had been inspired to do so after a visit to the Shanti Project, the San Francisco AIDS hospice which grew out of a gay men's spiritual circle in the 1980s.) After several years of successful work and growth, it is now the largest such hospice in Thailand, and a focus for donations from the concerned middle and upper classes of the area. It is a beautiful facility, and it offers people in need of pastoral and physical solace a peaceful and meditative refuge. Hundreds of Thais have died there, and hundreds more live there now.

In Chiang Mai, things were not as easy for Phra Pongthep, the activist monk who began the city's first AIDS refuge. Phra Pongthep is an unusual man by any measure. He is outspoken and direct, openly critical in a manner many Thais find unnerving. He pushes. When he first conceived of the idea of starting a hospice, the Abbot of his *wat* was strongly opposed. Phra Pongthep simply moved out, to what was essentially a shed near the main *wat*, and began. At first, patients slept in the open air, cared for only by Phra Pongthep and a few volunteers. He persisted, gradually building up the facility through donations. Kai Kawila Army Hospital donated beds and bedding. The Australian Government offered money for food and drugs. A taxi driver with HIV infection offered himself and his car to serve as a makeshift ambulance. Still-well people with HIV volunteered to help with the sick. A Dutch nurse spent several months training these volunteers. The place still looks more like a barn than a hospice, and it is nothing if not simple. It is always filled to capacity and over. Phra Pongthep, however, is not interested in expansion. He firmly believes that people with AIDS, as with any other illness, should be cared for at home. He is blunt with family members seeking to 'drop off' a sick relative. The people at his center are those without families, with nowhere else to go. If a family is at all able, Phra Pongthep works with them to care for their ill member, and offers the blessing and support which Thais find in their monks. Though a small and slender man, and young by Thai standards for a monk on his own (he is 35), he is a formidable figure, and compels his listeners with a sharp tongue and quick wit. He is also something of a radical, for many of the people dying at his small center are women, and he has, on occasion, to touch them (when lifting, for example, or checking the progress of a wound). Thai Buddhist tradition is notably conservative on this point: women and monks never have even the slightest physical contact. Women must stand on two legs, never one, in the presence of monks. A woman's laundry may not touch a monk. Phra Pongthep was challenged on the unorthodox nature of his work, and gave this answer:[1]

> Let me tell you a story. Soon after the passing of the Buddha, one of his disciples was walking toward Benares with a young novice. The two monks came to the River Jamuna, which was high after the rains. There was no boat, and they would have to walk across, using sticks. On the shore they found a young woman, stranded, who was too weak to make her way across. The novice was shocked when his old master picked up the woman, put her on his back, and carried her across to the far shore. Once across, the master put her down, and the two monks went on their way. The master said nothing about the event, but the novice was deeply disturbed. That night, he challenged the master: 'How could you have done such a thing?' To which the master replied, 'I only carried her across the river. You have carried her all the way here.'

The other strand of AIDS activism in Thailand, and one which is very much at the center of HIV/AIDS work in Cambodia, has grown out of women's movements in both countries, out of those groups concerned with the rights of women in the sex industry. When HIV hit Thailand, the only organizations already active with women in the sex trade were groups like EMPOWER, an NGO begun by Thai women to assist sex workers in Bangkok, and the Women's Relief Center, a safe-house for battered women run by a Thai Buddhist nun, Mae Chi Khunying Khanitta. The same holds true for the Cambodian Women's Development Association, which began as a women's rights body, took up the plight of trafficked sex workers, and is now one of the leading indigenous groups working on HIV prevention and care. These are all service organizations, whose mandates have had to change as HIV overwhelmed the women they were working with.

EMPOWER has the strengths and limitations inherent in the eclectic world of NGOs. It is small, with two offices: one in Bangkok and one in Chiang Mai. Its operating budget is correspondingly small. The group relies heavily on volunteers, and on larger donor agencies for providing the salaries of paid staff. The great strength of an organization like EMPOWER is not its scale, but its grassroots base – the women they work with know them intimately, trust them, share their lives with them. Jackie Pollock, an English teacher, has been with EMPOWER for over a decade, and helped found the Chiang Mai branch. Walking into a local brothel with Jackie is a lesson in the kind of relationships such commitment can build. If you step in as a man alone you'll see women and girls sitting around like rabbits: blank stares, little talk, faces flat and vague. When these same women see Jackie they burst into life, instantly becoming themselves – village girls again, full of warmth, hugging and laughing and talking. They love her, and in the loveless life of a sex worker, such human connections may be one of the few ties to hope.

EMPOWER began working with women in the sex trade well before HIV spread in Thailand. Now, about the half the women they work with have HIV, and many are beginning to progress to AIDS, and to die. What began as a service organization committed to empowering sex workers now has to cope with getting women (often illegal residents – about half are from Burma) medical care, and safe places to convalesce, and to pass. It is a sad reality of Thai medicine that sex workers generally get very poor care. They are rarely treated with respect, if they get any treatment at all. Once

HIV-infected, they get even less, their treatable symptoms dismissed as 'just a part of AIDS'. With an EMPOWER nurse along for their clinic visits or hospitalizations, they at least have an advocate. In the Thai context this is invaluable. Even the poorest of the poor are treated differently if they have a patron. If the patron is a foreigner, all the better.

Social activism of this kind is tolerated only with the strictest of government controls in the three communist states of the region, China, Laos, and Vietnam. Advocates for social or political change in these countries are routinely jailed, put in labor camps, or they disappear. China's treatment of dissidents is well known. Vietnam, despite its recent 'opening' to capitalist markets, is not much better; the Vietnamese regime continues to hold in prison senior Buddhist monks and Catholic priests who have resisted Communist Party control of their institutions. The 75-year-old Abbot of one of the country's principal Buddhist monasteries had his imprisonment extended another four years (to a total of eight) in 1996. His crime? Having assisted flood victims without permission from the Party. When I asked one of his disciples why he thought this 'crime' was being punished so harshly, he had this to say:

It is a question of ideology. The Party in power here believes in Marxist–Leninist–Maoist ideology. They cannot accept that Buddhism sees man differently. They are afraid of the peoples' love for our teacher here, and so they jail him. Actually, this is very irrational. If you take what people want away, try to destroy it, they will want it more. But our problem now is that our teacher is a very old man, and he is not well. They have denied us any real teaching here, and he is taken from us. So our Buddhist traditions are not being preserved and transmitted. I believe this regime will change, but by then it may be too late.

The price of social activism in Southeast Asia is high. In Burma, from 1962 until today, those Burmese who have challenged the successive military regimes have risked harassment, exile, prison, torture, extra-judicial execution, and the persecution of their families and contacts. That so many people have been willing to pay this price for so long is a testament to how deep the yearning for justice can be, how compelling the thirst for freedom. While superficially more law-abiding and progressive countries such as Thailand and Malaysia would seem to be safer for dissenters, both have exiled, jailed, and killed social activists with impunity. Seven people were assassinated in the build-up to Thailand's 1996 national elections. Labor and environmental leaders have been murdered, including the activist leader of The Forum for the Poor, a farmers' lobby that was trying to prevent a dam project from forcing the relocation of farming families in Thailand's impoverished northeast. In 1995 a community hospice for people with AIDS was fire-bombed in Thailand. Malaysia has jailed most of the leaders of a conservative Muslim political movement there, and is now actively pursuing charges against an advocate for illegal workers, Irene Fernandez, who exposed incidents of torture of Indonesian workers held in Malaysian detention centers.

AIDS activism in Southeast Asia has thus far not pushed for political reform; its focus has been on relatively less threatening calls for an end to discrimination, access to care, and dignity in death. As the numbers of affected persons begin to swell (which we know they will, since millions are already HIV-positive, though asymptomatic), this may change. Given the current political climate for dissent, AIDS activists in Asia are likely to face regimes sorely tested by their demands. AIDS activism may challenge and invigorate Buddhist movements as well. His Holiness the Dalai Lama of Tibet has called on the Buddhist clergy to become more engaged in worldly problems, citing the Christian clergy's involvement with liberation theology as an example of what Buddhism must do to stay relevant and alive. Maha Ghosananda has echoed this call for the Cambodian clergy. Nowhere has it been more strongly taken to heart than in Burma, where monks and nuns marched for democracy in their tens of thousands, and where abbots, teachers, and scholars of the Buddhist tradition languish in prisons and work on chain gangs. How many committed monks and nuns like Phra Pongthep are there in the prisons of Burma, Vietnam, and China?

Note

1. As told to Mr Anthony Niranam.

Part Three
Relativity and Culture

Why have we not responded? Working at one of the nation's finest academic institutions, I have sought advice from faculty colleagues in American history, law, and public health as to why our national response to the AIDS epidemic has been so inadequate. I have tried to find out what it is about our past that makes it so difficult for us to deal rationally with an epidemic of a fatal sexually transmitted disease. Two things are apparent. First, as a nation we have never 'conquered the Victorian within ourselves', preferring to deny our sexual behavior even when the behavior presents an untold risk to ourselves and our loved ones. Second, because HIV infection is contagious and presumed fatal, and AIDS is a disfiguring illness at its end stage that elicits fears about our own mortality, we have stigmatized AIDS and those populations with high rates of HIV infection. It is especially unfortunate that many of those infected have been from populations already stigmatized because of sexual orientation, race, occupation (e.g. sex workers), or other behavior (e.g. injecting drug use).

Michael H Merson, 'Returning home: reflections on the USA's response to the HIV/AIDS epidemic', Lancet, 1996.

19. Drug wars and the war on drugs

War and the social chaos and upheavals it brings make an almost ideal setting for epidemic diseases (from the Greek *epi demos*, 'upon the people'). There are no more moving descriptions of the toll these diseases exact than Walt Whitman's. The poet served as a field nurse in several military hospitals during the American Civil War and later published his war remembrances in *Specimen Days*, an unjustly neglected classic of his prose. Whitman watched young man after young man die of typhoid, burn out with fevers, waste away from diarrhea, and endure the miserable end of gangrene and repeated amputations – diseases for which treatment was almost non-existent at the time. The losses were immense, and because it was a civil war, all were ours. Among the soldiers, but particularly among women and children, malnutrition compounded the threat of epidemic diseases. Combine these threats, and war always does combine them, and it becomes clear that more people, and usually more civilians, lose their lives to breakdowns in food distribution, sanitation, and basic health care than to bullets, bombs, or executions. This appears to have been the case during the Khmer Rouge period: while 500,000 people are thought to have been murdered, another 1.5 million Cambodians are thought to have died of malnutrition, disease, and exhaustion from overwork.

For the modern West, epidemics of cholera or typhus, of death from gangrene and staph infections, are a part of distant memory, horrors of historical interest. But most 'modern' wars (and it need hardly be said that the scores of conflicts raging or simmering today are largely civil wars) are fought in field conditions no better than those of 19th-century America. You don't find antibiotics for typhoid fever in the Sudan, or disposable surgical equipment in the jungles of Burma; soldiers lose legs, and civilians die, in the same squalor and pain as they did on the battlefields of the American civil war. Health conditions in the Rwandan conflict were more like Old Testament-era pestilence and made 1860s Virginia look modern. The Hutu prisoners accused of genocide, an estimated 90,000 persons, are now housed in prisons so crowded and filthy that many are losing their feet and legs from a life of standing in pooled human feces and urine several feet deep. For the people of Somalia, Zaire/Congo, Khmer Rouge-controlled Cambodia, and the Shan states today, modern medical advances might as well have happened on the moon.

An early slogan of AIDS prevention campaigns in the US was 'AIDS does not discriminate'. While a useful battle cry, this is unfortunately only partly true. AIDS does discriminate: HIV spreads fastest where social life is chaotic, where poverty is endemic, where women are uneducated, and where the rights of vulnerable groups and individuals are violated. This is true in the world's poorest and most strife-torn nations, and it is true among the poor of rich nations, such as the US, where HIV spread continues to be localized in pockets of poverty and social disruption, our urban 'war zones', as they are sometimes called, the front line of our war on drugs. Civil war is perhaps the extreme case of social disruption; human rights violations are part and parcel of these conflicts, and so it may be only logical that HIV/AIDS should discriminate against peoples caught in the throes of civil strife. This may sound an uncommon interaction, but civil war and its social and health consequences are anything but uncommon in our time. HIV is only one of many infections that spread rapidly when social orders are chaotic, blood is being spilled, and women raped. But unlike cholera, which so devastated the Rwandan refugees, or malaria, which decimates the freedom fighters of Burma, HIV, with its stealthy incubation and trivial first symptoms, does not fit the usual mode of war-related disease outbreaks. To use a military analogy, cholera goes off like a cluster bomb; HIV seeds a country like land-mines, an analogy of painful aptitude for Cambodia.

Aside from the direct impact of civilian casualties in war (including land-mines), the social disruption of civil unrest can be fertile ground for more complex health effects. The list of countries where spread of HIV has been facilitated by political repression, social disruption, and civil strife is long, and includes at least Uganda in the 1970s and 1980s, Zaire, Kenya, Rwanda, Burundi, and Haiti. Could the argu-

ment be turned around as well? Could the loss to AIDS of heads of
households, wage earners, the educated and traveling adults of these
countries be a component cause of social disruption, of chaos? This
is perhaps an impossible question to answer. But these losses, and the
burdens they place on society are going to plague places like Burma
and Cambodia, if and when they finally find peace.

A twist of the civil conflict currently tearing Burma apart is that
the war is intimately connected to the heroin trade. It has been labeled
a 'drug war,' with all the negative implications such a label carries.
This was also the case in Afghanistan and Lebanon, where drugs
bought munitions, and where the porous borders and lawlessness of
long-standing conflict made narcotics trafficking comparatively easy.
War is good for the drug business, the return of civil society and the
rule of law a problem. The black-market cash-flows that drugs generate enrich and empower just those anti-democratic and violent
elements who then have a stake in seeing civil conflicts continue. This
forces insurgents into a Faustian bargain: they need guns, and may
have to allow narcotics production to get them, but this very process
undermines their aims, if these should be, as in the case of the Shans
and Wa, the defeat of an oppressive military junta and a return to
civilian rule. Once a conflict is labeled a 'drug war', the international
community shuns it; the media often pull out as well, all other
elements of the struggle are subsumed under the rubric of 'narco-
terrorism' or 'drug warlordism'. This has been the enduring tragedy
of the Shan people: since their leaders have been implicated in heroin
production, their aspirations have been trivialized. Civilians in this
conflict get no support in the UN or from relief agencies. The Hmong
in Laos, just across the border, are caught in a similar quandary. Their
struggle has been reduced by observers to a 'drug conflict', and their
legitimate grievances against the Lao belittled. They too are alone.

The heroin trade starts, of course, with farmers.[1] In the case of
the Shan, Wa, Kachin, and Hmong, these are subsistence farmers,
peasants and civilians. Of the immense revenues their opium crops
generate, they see only pennies. The farmers of these hidden hills
might do better for their families growing coffee or tea, grain or
cotton. But the men with the guns, from both rebel and national
armies, want them – in some areas force them – to grow poppies.
Billions of dollars a year come out of these hills, and the ordinary
people are in rags. Those with energy and courage try to escape, to

find work in Thailand, where much of the profit is laundered, invested, and goes on to generate more wealth. But not for them; they
just build the buildings.

The Swedish researcher and author Bertil Lintner, and his wife, a
Shan social activist, are undoubtedly the leading experts on the
complex narcotics industry in Burma, on its political roots and
implications. In his encyclopedic study *Burma in Revolt: Opium and
Insurgency since 1948*, Lintner argues convincingly that the narcotics
trade in Burma cannot be understood outside the context of the
civil war, and that only a political solution in the Shan and Wa states
can possibly lead to a reduction in opium dependency. He stresses
that the narcotics control agencies in the west active in Burma
(including the US Drug Enforcement Agency, the DEA) have focused
almost entirely on criminalizing the trade, seeing it somehow as an
aberration, and not as an intrinsic component of both the insurgents
and the military. The logical outcome of the DEA approach would
be to offer assistance to Burma's narcotics control program, which
the US has done in the past. The problem with this, Lintner argues,
is that the junta, or people within it, are also involved. Strengthening
them may do no more than increase their market share of the heroin
trade, and empower them in the war against the Shans. Whatever
we may think about this argument, recent events in Burma would
suggest that Lintner is correct in his assertion. The most powerful
leader in the Shan states for much of the last 15 years was a man
named Khun Sa, also known as Chang Chifu, a Chinese–Shan
warlord. His Mong Tai Army (MTA) once had 15,000 well-armed
fighters, and controlled a significant portion of the Shan states. His
insurgency was widely known to be supported on Shan opium,
though he also controlled several lucrative jade mines. Khun Sa was
labeled US enemy number one by the DEA. House leaders like
Representative Charlie Rangel of New York, concerned about the
devastation heroin was bringing to his district (Harlem), asked for
lethal aid for the DEA and SLORC to capture Khun Sa and bring
him to justice. But in early 1996, in a surprise move that threw the
Shan states (and US policy) into disarray, Khun Sa 'surrendered' to
the SLORC. The US State Department immediately called for his
extradition to stand trial for narcotics trafficking, and publicly offered
SLORC a US$2-million ransom for him. SLORC refused; (US$2
million, considering that Khun Sa reportedly ran as much as one-

third of the world's heroin business, is an almost laughable sum – we are talking here about wealth on another scale). Instead, the *New Light of Myanmar*, SLORC's mouthpiece, began referring to Khun Sa as U Khun Sa, signifying a respected elder. SLORC and U Khun Sa have now embarked on a joint-venture bus company.

There have been no winners in this tango, but many losers. The DEA loses credibility throughout the region, as it is once again confirmed that they 'don't get it'. Harlem loses. But no one has suffered more than the Shans. Many supported Khun Sa because of his populist, Shan nationalist rhetoric. He was supposed to be fighting SLORC, and leading the Shans toward independence, or at least autonomy within a federal union. He sold his people to SLORC without their permission and without warning. Two factions split from the MTA over the surrender, led by commanders who wanted to keep the Shan resistance alive. SLORC, however, quickly overran the Shan states. Three-way fighting soon broke out between the SLORC, the Wa, and the Lahu in the Shan states – a land grab/drug war/criminal enterprise that further ravaged the Shans. The farmers of the hills are still growing opium at gunpoint, though who for is less clear, and massive population transfers are underway throughout the region, an attempt on SLORC's part to isolate the rebels still fighting. More Shans are migrating to Thailand, more women and girls are being trafficked into the sex trade, the war widens and deepens, HIV spread continues unchecked, and U Khun Sa is reportedly living in Rangoon, along the same lakefront avenue as Ne Win. Dictators in retirement seem to get less ideological.

Spill-overs of the Burma–Laos heroin trade are causing problems for other countries in the region, notably India and China. The road leading out of the western Chin hills and into India's frontier state of Manipur carries opium out by the truckload. Manipur, closed to the world through years of ethnic insurgency, now has one of India's worst heroin addiction problems, and among the highest HIV rates of any state in the country. Ethnic peoples on both sides of this border are heavily affected, and heroin is reaching India's cities and her youth. The Burmese spill-over into China, as discussed in the section on China, amounted to perhaps 80% of China's entire HIV burden in 1996, making control of Burma's heroin trade an issue of national importance for China as well as for India. But China's position is murky.

The region's heroin cartels are reported to be largely controlled by ethnic Chinese clans. These, historically, were outgrowths of the Chinese Nationalist forces (Kuomintang – KMT) that remained trapped in Yunnan and Burma when Chiang Kai Shek fled to Taiwan after his defeat by Mao and the Communists. Old links and clan ties have remained, and seemingly outlasted ideological conflicts. The opium grown in Burma and Laos, and refined in Laos, moves via Kunming to Shanghai, Hong Kong, and then to the West, where it is sold. The picture emerges of a new opium war, but one inverted from the 19th-century opium war which so devastated China. In the earlier conflict, India was the farmland for opium; the British were the cartel, carrying opium to China's ports. Britain made an immense fortune from the revenue, which was invested in London. China was humiliated, weakened, and impoverished. Now the cartels are Chinese, the markets in the West, and the cities rising to new heights on the revenues are Shanghai and Kunming. Poetic justice, perhaps, but in both opium wars the casualties are high, the money stained with blood.

The War on Drugs, as opposed to these drug wars, has given us another set of problems. First and foremost, the US has failed to fulfil its end of the bargain – reducing demand. Heroin in 1996 is more plentiful, cheaper, and more powerful than at any time in the past. It has replaced cocaine in many settings as the major hard drug of abuse. We have jailed hundreds of thousands of Americans to no avail. Drug treatment lags in research, in effectiveness, and in scope. And, as we've discussed, the HIV preventive measures that could reduce the harm of heroin use, like needle exchanges, have proven almost impossible to mount in America, which continues to see drug use as criminal behavior, deserving punishment more than treatment. The War on Drugs has been as manifest a failure as our DEA policies in Burma. In both cases, the suffering that has ensued as a result of these failures is immense. Are there other approaches, however politically unfeasible in the current climate of opinion?

Without a political settlement to the Burmese civil war, Burma will continue to export increasing quantities of heroin (output has doubled since 1988 alone, according to US DEA reports). SLORC's treatment of U Khun Sa has shown that they cannot be expected to resolve the problem – they are in too deep. China may have a conflict of interest in seeing a stable, prosperous Burma. ASEAN, India,

Europe, Japan and the US should recognize these realities and use all pressure available, including economic sanctions, to bring about tri-partite negotiations in Burma. To bring to the table SLORC, the National League for Democracy, and the ethnic nationalities for substantive resolutions of the deadlock. This is what the elected leaders have called for since 1990, as has the UN in its annual affirmation of the standing resolution calling for the restoration of democracy. Until such talks start, and begin to yield real progress, further investment in the SLORC is supporting the heroin trade – it is as simple as that. And so the oil companies Unocal and Total are supporting the heroin trade, however indirectly, and undermining the Burmese people's chances for peace.

Crop substitution programs, supported by the US, have proven quite successful in decreasing opium production in Thailand, now no longer a significant grower. Part of the success of this program, undoubtedly, was the openness and transparency of the Thai state to US officials, researchers, and even tourists, in the hills. With a political resolution in Burma, and greater openness in Laos, these approaches might succeed again. Significant development funds from donor agencies are also certainly going to be needed to help develop viable alternative economies.

If the current crop were reduced by half, there would be about 30% less heroin in the US market coming from the golden triangle. What effect would that have? Opium growing is already spreading in Mexico and central America, where the cartels have introduced the poppy as a new cash crop. If demand remained unchanged, wouldn't the growers simply go elsewhere? What about Tajikistan or Azerbaijan, which have the requisite social chaos and insurgency? Very little research is being done on the treatment of opiate addiction. Methadone is an old and imperfect treatment, but one of the few agents in use. We urgently need research into new and better treatment methods, and into drug prevention programs that work. A two-pronged attack of reduced supply (and therefore greater cost) and better treatment might make a real dent in the heroin problems of the United States and Europe.

In the meantime, HIV-preventive measures, such as needle exchange, need to be implemented broadly; needle exchange can also help get addicts into treatment, a rare win–win in our losing war on drugs.

Note

1. Buying the raw opium crop from these farmers is cheap, orders of magnitude less expensive then trying to intercept processed heroin further down the pipeline. During the Carter administration the concept of simply buying the Shan opium crop (then it would have cost about US$10 million) was openly discussed. The policy was called 'preemptive purchase' and had been developed by Carter's special advisor on health, Peter Bourne. It was extremely unpopular in some circles, hailed in others. Serious discussion of the plan was terminated when Peter Bourne was photographed, infamously, using cocaine at an official function. He was dismissed from the White House, and the plan went with him. The Wa are still interested, and have been pressing for direct sales of their crops to the US Drug Enforcement Agency (DEA) for the past eight years; they have no interest in supporting addiction in the US, and are seeking support for their cause. We are not buying, however, preferring to spend many hundreds of millions more on trying to stop heroin imports after the cartels have the drugs. This outcome is so illogical as to be perverse, but from a policy perspective perhaps unavoidable, and from a DEA perspective, essential to the survival of their expansive law enforcement budgets.

20. Medical ethics, human rights, Asian values

AIDS-related human rights activism, sharing the orientation of mainstream human rights, has focused on the visible and purposeful governmental acts that jeopardize individual privacy, liberty, and protection against discrimination. Human rights obligations stemming from the right to health care, to social assistance, or from the necessity to improve the enjoyment of human rights through international co-operation have been neglected.

AIDS in the World

Civil society, the intricate network of shared rights and responsibilities, of social contracts and the integrity of persons, the customs and ways which make a people and a culture, is a living entity. Century-slow beings rise out of time and human interaction, each with its own peculiar vitality. A civil society is a being made by countless individuals, past and present. It lives in that most fragile of abodes, the collective hearts of a populace, in memory, presence, and hope. Precisely because it is so much the creation of a people, civil culture is at once beautifully resilient and deeply vulnerable. A functioning civil society is something like an old-growth forest, full of hidden networks and balances, sustainable and generative. Because the maintenance of civility requires human input, it is perhaps more a garden than a forest, a garden that requires constant care to bring out the inherent beauty of its plantings, and to create spaces of peace, reflection and inspiration. Like a garden, civil culture too has its wild untended corners, its secret places, secluded corners for lovers and sunlit benches for the old. A Pol Pot, a Ne Win with a band of thugs, an army of Red Guards, can devastate the exquisite gardens of a people with frightening speed and consequences. Sarajevo was once a model of what the Balkans might become: multi-ethnic, sophisticated, tolerant, handsome.

Nowhere is the death of a civil culture more jarring than in China today. What the 11-year cultural revolution did not destroy is now threatened by a drive for wealth so intense that you literally choke on its fumes. And this in China, where the orientation of man to his culture and fellows evolved into a kind of secular faith in humanity, ripened over three millennia of carefully recorded history. You see the destruction of civil culture everywhere in the Middle Kingdom, in the garishness of modern Chinese 'traditional' arts (historical references as kitsch, greeting-card Buddhas, hopelessly tacky dragons festooning every overworked surface), the crudeness of social interaction, the brutality of its politics, the suppression of ideas and the degradation of the environment. Yet China looks sane and functional when compared with Burma and Cambodia, where civil society is still a shambles.

Burma and Cambodia have no common border. What they do share, in addition to ancient, profound Buddhist traditions and past periods of great cultural achievement, are political cultures marked by state violence and corruption, chronic civil war and insurgency, and explosive recent epidemics of HIV infection. It seems almost unbearable that the peoples of these troubled lands should have to face yet another lethal set of obstacles to peace, national reconciliation, and health. But an examination of global HIV/AIDS epidemiology in the developing world suggests that their situations may be not atypical. Uganda in the recent past could be used to make the same argument, as could Haiti under the chaotic military rule of General Cedras; these are countries that have shared the misfortune of having HIV ravage their populations during periods of civil strife under incompetent governments, when civil society was profoundly endangered.

There is no doubt that promotion of condom use is a more direct intervention target than, say, the ending of a simmering insurgency or the establishment of a free press. However, it is perhaps also true that without some measure of social stability and respect for human rights and freedoms, targeted interventions of the sort currently being promoted (condom use, better STD care, HIV education for youths) may not be sustainable. This is particularly true for prevention programs aimed at women, who universally suffer most when the civic order is chaotic and violent. Such programs may have more problematic consequences as well.

Foreign aid, development assistance, and technical support have all been necessary to help poor countries contend with HIV/AIDS. These programs, however, can also serve to support problematic regimes and leaders, principally by lending international legitimacy to regimes in power. Governments whose policies could be argued to have hindered HIV prevention or worsened its spread could include Burma's junta, the Ceaucescu regime in Romania, Mobuto Sese Seko's single-party state in Zaire, the apartheid government of South Africa, and several successive regimes in Rwanda. Supporting such regimes, and lending them legitimacy through donation of HIV/AIDS moneys, may assist in prolonging the political and social situations that have led to explosive HIV spread. The Burmese junta is actively seeking such legitimacy, and defended itself in the December 1995 UN hearings on human rights violations in the country by listing the number of international agencies and NGOs collaborating with them on HIV/AIDS programs, among others. While researchers and prevention experts may bear no ill intent, and indeed may struggle to establish ethical standards for their own projects in countries like Burma, there are larger ethical issues at stake. Burma has lost so many of her health professionals, educators, and civil servants, not because of poverty or lack of support for social programs, but through repression, imprisonment, and murder. The junta itself has helped create the lack of needed professionals. To support such regimes, particularly, as Aung San Suu Kyi has said, when we ourselves come from countries which tolerate basic freedoms and human rights, is, if we accept this premise, illogical in itself, whatever 'good' we believe we are doing by our presence.

A new paradigm for understanding the relationships of public health problems and political realities may be required if we are to address challenges like the spread of HIV/AIDS in countries in turmoil. While humanitarian assistance and strict ethical standards for international involvement must remain priorities, the integration of human rights and political realities into public health discourses and analyses is needed. At the last Asia–Pacific meeting on AIDS, a call was made to 'de-politicize' AIDS. Perhaps the precise opposite approach is called for: to recognize and attempt to respond to the crucial impact political and social realities have on the dynamics of this, and other, diseases. For many countries there may be no more effective HIV-prevention program than the respect for human rights that comes with peace.

The interaction of HIV, political instability, and human rights abuses in places like Burma, Cambodia, Romania and Zaire should not be surprising; social resources for public health are limited in these countries even in peacetime; their governments are all too often incompetent, corrupt, or both, and persecution against minority groups, intellectuals, journalists, and educated elites are commonplace. Yet in the now extensive HIV/AIDS literature these political realities are too rarely included in discussions of epidemiology, national vulnerability, or barriers to prevention. We are more likely to be informed that in a war-torn African country (several could be named) lack of male circumcision has facilitated HIV spread than that government censorship has eroded a free press, rape of women is widespread and largely unpunished, or that donor funds for health programs have been squandered by corrupt or inept officials. Measures of risk in the public-health literature typically focus exclusively on the behaviors of individuals, even in settings where social systems are patent obstacles to risk reduction. This is not only a lack of intellectual honesty on the part of the medical community, it is bad science.

The classical unit of analysis in epidemiology has been the individual HIV seroconverter and her or his risks. From the behaviors associated with HIV seroconversion, we deduce trends in risk groups, and, if our studies have enough power, in larger populations. This approach has its strengths (rigor, precision, ease of analysis) but also profound limitations. Epidemiology should, at its best, guide and focus preventive efforts. If political and social factors in a given country hinder prevention efforts or facilitate the spread of HIV, these root causes should logically be part of research efforts and intervention programs. Such factors are seldom considered in publications in the medical literature, those of my group included. If they are not included, countries where epidemic spread of HIV is under way are unlikely to achieve control. Yet the public health community is concerned with human rights, particularly as regards the rights of individuals with HIV/AIDS. The foci of these concerns, however, have traditionally been quite narrow. We have paid considerable attention to the ethics of HIV-testing and counseling, informed consent procedures, discrimination and confidentiality, forced or *de facto* isolation and confinement of HIV infected persons, access to care, and the rights of research subjects. There is a large literature around these issues, and articulated systems of review to ensure ethical and human rights standards are met, particularly in research. This is laudable, and by no means to be diminished in importance. But without a wider examination of the human rights context of public health programs, these parameters may be so narrow as to have little actual impact. In Burma, citizens are denied freedom of speech or assembly, a free press, and the right to vote, to create independent non-governmental organizations, and to criticize the junta and its policies. Arbitrary arrest, incarceration without trial, and extra-judicial execution by SLORC have all been documented. Can the rights of people with AIDS be addressed in any meaningful way without taking into account the wider reality of human rights under this regime? To phrase the question differently: can a political body with such policies be expected either to respect the rights of people with or without HIV/AIDS, or to enact effective HIV/AIDS programs?

Perhaps the position of Archbishop Desmond Tutu during the apartheid struggle in South Africa best illustrates where AIDS researchers and organizations eager to help the Burmese people find themselves. Tutu opposed the immunization programs Unicef wanted to mount in the old South Africa. Unicef's position was that 'children are above politics'. Tutu's was that the apartheid system, not lack of vaccines, was at the root of the disproportionate mortality among black children. Since Unicef's involvement would give legitimacy to the apartheid government's claims to be 'helping' blacks, it had to be resisted. The test of this stance may not be the absolutist moral position that helping children is always a good, but the more complex reality that anything which sustains evil (even medical aid) may prolong suffering. Unicef is now active in post-apartheid South Africa. It remains to be seen if their partnership with the Mandela regime, and those that come after it, can reduce preventable mortality among South Africa's children. But at the very least there is now a government in power with some accountability, a government that can be openly challenged in elections if it fails, which was not the case under apartheid, where Unicef's successes or failures would have been closed to scrutiny, as they now are under SLORC.

Human rights and Asian values

Are the human rights enshrined in the UN charter and the Geneva Accords applicable in countries like Burma, Indonesia, Malaysia,

Vietnam, and China (all of which have argued that they are not)? Or are they imposed by a hostile West on competitor states who have the right to their own interpretation of human rights, which may radically differ from the 'international standard'? Central to the current debate on economic and trade policies and human rights between Asia and the West has been a focus on 'Traditional Asian Values' as opposed to Western ones. Crudely defined (and it is a crude debate, at best), the discourse posits that the Pacific Rim political systems place collective values over individual freedoms, the right to grow economically over the right to express dissent, and the duties and obligations of fixed and reciprocal Confucian hierarchies over democratic principles, including liberal notions of privacy and individuality. Asian economies are growing in the double digits, so the defenders of these values suggest, because Asians are obedient and thrifty; the family, not the State, insures the elderly and the infirm; long-lasting and stable governments ensure long-term planning. The failures of development schemes in Africa and Central America can be seen, in this rubric, to be failures of *values*, Asian miracles as successful examples of the Asian 'way'. These miracle states have also succeeded, so the argument goes, by active suppression of the 'decadent' aspects of modernity, while favoring culturally appropriate expressions of nationalism. Western leaders and the business community, which perhaps belongs to neither East nor West, have understandably begun to support these notions. The dismantling of government social programs across Europe and the US is being accomplished through accepting these values as a challenge to the West's notions of the role of government and the need to compete. It is only natural that business leaders would find appealing the idea that trade unions should be government-controlled, as in Indonesia and China, or that environmental safeguards should never inhibit economic growth, a situation that has already severely damaged the ecosystems of Taiwan, Thailand, China, and others, and that workers should be poorly paid, as they are almost right across Asia. For governments too, the concept that expensive social programs should be scrapped in favor of 'family values' has its appeal. And what government, East or West, would not like to have its exports delinked from any consideration of health, safety, workers' rights, or environmental impacts? Add an open market in weapons and you have a recipe for unprecedented global economic growth.

This can sound like the blueprint for a new era of global prosperity and free trade, or a deeply threatening scenario which could logically include the destruction of the global environment, the end of workers' rights worldwide, an arms race in Asia, and the acceptance of authoritarian government and corporate irresponsibility as viable alternatives to democracy and the rule of law. While the democratic states of the West will no doubt continue to hold elections, have something like a free press, and maintain some aspects of social programs, the need to compete with countries without these restraints on governments and companies would make real opposition virtually impossible. If market forces and unelected governments alone determine the policies of a country, the rights and choices of citizens will be very much beside the point. This is why, while we should perhaps not expect much challenge to the current flirtation with 'Asian values' from the corporate sector, or from governments in power, we should certainly be hearing from citizens' groups, intellectuals, the media, and others who have an interest in people's rights to determine what kind of country, and what kind of world, they want to live in. But the authoritarian governments (China, Indonesia, Malaysia, Burma, Vietnam, and Laos, to name a few) who embrace and promote the concepts of Asian values, do not allow these voices to be heard. The price for dissent in such countries is extraordinarily high. When protests are raised by Western voices, 'neo-colonialism' is invoked, or interference in the internal affairs of a sovereign state.

Aung San Suu Kyi has penetrated the moral morass of 'Asian values' with characteristic candor and insight. In a videotaped address to the International Labor Organization in Manila in 1995, she pointed out that the rhetoric of the universal rights of man was a cornerstone of Asia's independence movements at the end of the colonial period. Nehru, Sukarno, her father Aung San, and Bandaranaike of Sri Lanka all insisted that Asians should have the same rights as Europeans, rights that been explicitly denied them under European rule. The new states of the region have enshrined these independence heroes in their pantheons, and invoke their names in the search for legitimacy. These new elites, however, have found colonial-era restrictions on democratic rule, dissent, and basic freedoms too tempting and too profitable to ignore. They now insist that their countries have no tradition of universal values, that these are western impositions, not the very bases of their respective states.

Aung San would shudder in horror to discover that the military he founded has perpetuated colonial harshness while eroding what useful legacies the British did leave behind: educational institutions, basic infrastructure, a working public health system.

Given the chance, the people of Burma did not choose 'Asian values'. In the 1990 elections, they chose the only voice Burma has for universal human rights, respect for the rights of citizens, and non-violent dissent: the National League for Democracy led by Aung San Suu Kyi. If the people of Indonesia, or of Vietnam or Laos, were offered a similar opportunity to choose, would they prefer 'Asian values' over the right to speak and think freely, the right to unionize? Until Asians have the right to vote on the 'Asian values' now promoted by their rulers, we should remain deeply skeptical about what unelected governments tell us their citizens want.

'Asian values' were a cornerstone of the thinking prevalent in the mid-1980s, which argued that Asia was spared an HIV problem because of her conservative mores. The decadent west and un-civilized Africans had 'values' problems, which Asians did not. This thinking has since been shown to have been hopelessly wrong-headed. 'Asian values' and traditions did, in fact, have a significant role to play in HIV, not as protective factors, but as risks. Traditions like prostitution, the trafficking and sale of women, the widespread use of these women by unmarried and married men alike, and the extreme reticence of wives to confront their husbands on these grounds, all served to sharply increase HIV susceptibility across the region. It is these traditions that have led to the ultimate violation of persons – slavery; in the Southeast Asian case, debt-bonded sexual slavery. Is there a clearer violation of the shared values of human beings than sex slavery?

Slavery and forced labor are components of the economic systems of Burma and China, and both have been 'censured' for these practices. They continue. In the case of Burma, the complaints have been louder, and there has been real divestment (Levi Strauss, Amoco, Liz Clairborne – a number of companies have pulled out of Burma). China is another matter; investment continues, and the US has neatly articulated how and why. We have 'delinked' human rights issues from trade issues in our dealings with the world's largest potential consumer market. With this sleight of hand we avoid some very complex realities, and we sell out those 1.3 billion consumers at the speed of the sound-bite. But, like a sound-bite, this is easier said than done; 'delinking' economics and human rights may be structurally impossible, in addition to being ethically obscene.

Trade between states is based, at the simplest level, on the economies of the states involved, and economies do not exist without people and their productivity. The conditions of a people, the ways in which their labor, or the resources of the land on which they live, generate wealth is the basis of any economy, and this is the context wherein human rights exist or are violated. Are the people slaves or free agents? If they are exploited by an elite, is the elite corrupt? Can it be held accountable? Are the people organized? Do they have a say in how their lands are used? Can they vote if they do not want their forest cleared or their river dammed? These are questions that cannot be answered without looking at economics and at rights. When people (take the Burmese, for example, or the Chinese who joined the students during the Tiananmen uprising) attempt to claim their rights, to insist that they have a say in how their country be run, basic economic relationships are inextricable from their other demands. The Chinese and Burmese democracy movements were as much protests against corruption and nepotism as they were movements for improvements in human rights. To then say, as the Clinton administration has said, that trade and human rights can be dealt with separately, that prison labor and the murder of activists can be neatly put aside when economic considerations are being discussed, is not only a wrong but an absurdity.

This absurdity is not lost on the elites in question. They have really only one concern: power and the privileges of power. As long as trade is uninterrupted, and investment in the economies under their control moves forward, what incentive is there to alter the conditions of that control? And if those conditions involve forced labor, population transfers, the movement of small farmers off their lands, the clear-cutting of forests, the suppression of dissent, why change any of this (profitable in the short term, if not the long) if investors are willing to go along? So the Finance Minister of the SLORC, Brigadier-General David Abel, could comment after another round of 'denunciations' and 'condemnations in the strongest possible language' of his regime in the UN, that, after all, business was still good and foreign investments moving ahead. And the US, loudest of all critics, still went ahead with the single largest infrastructure deal in the country, the Unocal oil and gas pipeline. This makes a mockery of the Burmese people's belief that the West – the US and the UN – cares about their rights.

The same complacency must be easing itself into the minds of China's politburo. They make a symbol of Wang Dan, sentencing him to 11 years in prison on the eve of an Asian summit with the US, not to insult Bill Clinton or unnerve Warren Christopher, but to remind their own people that trade and human rights are not connected in the 'New World Order', that they can expect no support from the West: that they are alone.

We should, perhaps, be more honest, if only not to delude the brave civilians facing these utterly ruthless elites. We should say, 'It is up to you to change things; we are only interested in the money your country brings to our country, and in the jobs at home our trade with you will help to generate and sustain. If you can seize the day, do it, but be prepared to continue our trade, or we will see to it that you don't get power.' If we really do care that the tennis shoes we buy are cheap because the hands that made them are in chains, we should not buy the shoes.

21. Democracy, empowerment, and health

People's participation in social and political transformation is the central issue of our time. This can only be achieved through the establishment of societies which place human worth above power, and liberation over control. In this paradigm, development requires democracy, the genuine empowerment of the people.

Aung San Suu Kyi, 'Empowerment for a Culture of Peace and Development', address to the World Commission on Culture and Development, Manila, 21 November 1994, delivered by Corazon Aquino.

The monsoon season of 1996 brought much more than rain to the people of Southeast Asia. After more than 30 years of authoritarian rule, Indonesians took to the streets in protest over a ban on the fledgling opposition led by Megawati Sukarnoputri, daughter of independence hero General Sukarno. The Suharto regime looked briefly, like its kingly head, mortal. Tellingly, Megawati's supporters marched through the streets of Jakarta carrying banners with two faces: Megawati's and Aung San Suu Kyi's. The military rulers of Burma and Indonesia may refuse to see connections between the democratic forces at work in their countries, but the people are far ahead of them.

In Cambodia, the Khmer Rouge leadership split over money matters (gem mining and logging concessions). Ieng Sary, Pol Pot's Minister for Foreign Affairs, asked for a royal pardon for his role in the deaths of more than a million people, in exchange for parting ways with his former colleague. He received his pardon in September, and a job in the government looked certain until Hun Sen's *coup d'état* in June 1997. Cambodia's democratic party leader, Sam Rainsy, was one of the few voices of dissent. Rainsy had been finance minister in the ruling coalition after the UN-sponsored general elections. He was known as the only non-corrupt member of the cabinet. One of the few issues that the dueling first and second prime ministers of this shaky coalition agreed upon was his dismissal. His integrity was an embarrassment to all concerned. When the co-prime ministers invited the SLORC Chairman, General Than Shwe, to Phnom Penh in October 1996, only Rainsy and his supporters protested (the French and British ambassadors to Cambodia went so far as to meet Than Shwe's flight). Intimidation and disappearances have thinned the ranks of his party, but Rainsy is undaunted, and has wide support among the people. In violent Cambodia, his life is daily in danger.

In May 1996, Aung San Suu Kyi, also under constant threat, called the first full congress of her party since her 1995 release. The junta arrested nearly all those planning to attend (that is, virtually all the country's elected leaders, more than 290 people). So far, three have died in detention, and several of those closest to Suu Kyi have been sentenced to 7–14 years in jail for 'sedition', and 'threatening the stability of the nation'. They were nearly all members of the 1990 parliament, which has yet to convene. A second party Congress in October led to 1,300 detentions and arrests, this time targeting the second tier of NLD leadership throughout the country, and the youth arm of the party. The junta is making headway in prohibiting the democratic process, and in ensuring that if the people of Burma do take to the streets, as they did in 1988, there will be no ability to organize the protests. They want a bloodbath to justify the need for military intervention and rule, and they may get one.

In Thailand, Prime Minister Banharn Silpa-Archa was forced out of office in October 1996 by a vote of no confidence stemming from a seemingly endless string of corruption charges, land scams, bank closures and indictments. The ensuing election season was marked by the worst violence, and the largest number of political assassinations, since the 1970s. After several years of mismanagement, the Thai economic boom is showing signs of bust, the country's credit rating has been downgraded on international markets, and Bangkok's seemingly insoluble problems (traffic, pollution, sprawl) continue to worsen.

In June 1996 Vietnam held its first full Communist Party Congress in several years, and closed the country as tight as in the old bamboo-curtain days, affecting not only investors' confidence, but thousands of small businessmen beginning to live off tourism revenues. The congress opted for stability rather than change, and their 'mini-boom' is also showing signs of stalling; investors complain about corruption, mismanagement, and party interference in decision-making. Many joint ventures never get off the ground; half of those that do fail.

And in this same tumultuous season, two East Timorese social activists shared the 1996 Nobel Peace Prize for their search for a peaceful resolution to Indonesia's occupation of their country. When they attempted to hold a conference in Malaysia on the plight of their homeland shortly after the prize was announced, the Prime Minister of Malaysia had them, and two Roman Catholic bishops, arrested and deported. He publicly stated that his reason for doing so was to avoid offending Indonesia's leaders.

The 1980s and 1990s have been times of extraordinary growth and change for Southeast Asia, an unprecedented period of economic growth for Thailand, Malaysia, Singapore and Indonesia; a protracted grappling with reform in the communist states of China, Laos and Vietnam; a painful and incomplete rebirth for Cambodia, deadlock and stagnation for Burma. Economic growth on the scale seen in some of these countries has demanded expansion in education, openness to the wider world, trade and more trade. These changes were meant, at least in the Thai case, to lead to a new era of empowerment for ordinary people, for democratization. But on this front, 1996 was an ominous year. New responses were not as forthcoming as old authoritarian habits; the leaders of Indonesia, Burma, and China responded to voices calling for change with the only tools they know – repression, arrests, state violence, rigidity. Old patterns of patronage, nepotism, and nationalism continue to undermine the effectiveness of these governments, to frustrate movements toward democracy, and to inhibit the kinds of social change that these countries urgently need if they are going to address the aspirations of their increasingly vocal peoples, the crises of their environments, and the regional HIV/AIDS crisis.

The links between empowerment, democracy, and health are neither abstract nor idealistic. When people have a say in political life, in setting national priorities, improvements in health and education are among their first objectives. This has been true in the US (George Bush was supposed to be the education president, Bill Clinton the health-care reformer and then preserver of Medicare) and it has been very much the case in Asia, where the hunger for educational opportunity is old and deep, as is the value given to good health and long life. But without government accountability, these highly valued social goods are difficult, even impossible, to achieve. And without democracy, accountability is a pipe dream. The Burma scholar Martin Smith has succinctly stated the relationship between democratic rights, censorship and health in his recent *Fatal Silence: Freedom of Expression and the Right to Health in Burma*:

> In a context of censorship and secrecy individuals cannot make informed decisions on important matters affecting their health. Without freedoms of academic research and ability to disseminate research findings, there can be no informed public debate. Denial of research and information also makes effective health planning and provision less likely at the national level. Without local participation, founded on freedom of expression and access to information, the health needs of many sections of society are likely to remain unaddressed. Likewise, secrecy and censorship have a negative impact on the work of international humanitarian agencies.

While Smith was referring specifically to Burma, his statements could be applied to any setting where lack of basic democratic freedoms can inhibit health and social programs. In the context of sexually transmitted diseases and drug use, many nations might fail the test of having truly informed public debates, access to information, and openness instead of secrecy.

What does the future hold for democratization in the region? ASEAN is now debating whether to admit Burma, and thus SLORC, into the regional forum.[1] They are under quiet but intense pressure from the US, the European Union, and Japan to delay this decision until there is some movement toward political resolution and respect for human rights in the country. Aside from SLORC's odious human rights record, there are other issues at stake. ASEAN wants to be seen as a 'safe' investment environment, as stable and prosperous. SLORC's corruption, drug revenue financing, and the inherent instability of the union under martial law make her an unappealing new member, at least in some quarters. But SLORC can deliver on other fronts. Burma has natural resources such as timber and jade, which have become rare in deforested Southeast Asia. There are all those untaxed US$20 bills to launder, and a banking system that might as well not exist, given the total lack of scrutiny surrounding it. And then there is the real prize: offshore oil and natural gas reserves, which are thought to be immense. These fields are under development, in a series of joint venture projects involving the SLORC, the French National Energy Corporation Total, and the California public company Unocal. ASEAN, quite logically, wants to be in on this deal. Thailand has already signed, and will be buying Burma's natural gas as soon as a pipeline (construction began in 1996) from the Gulf of Martaban, off Burma's southern coast, is completed. Western demands to respect human rights in Burma, and to delay entry into ASEAN until there are improvements, ring wildly false when French and American public companies are making multi-million-dollar investments in the junta. If past history (Nigeria, Ecuador) is any indicator, we should not expect an improvement in human rights or in health in Burma from the involvement of these giants. Should the junta be able to hold out against the people of Burma till oil revenues begin to flow, pushing for change will almost certainly become much more difficult.

Vietnam is already an ASEAN member; Laos and Cambodia are slated for ASEAN membership. The future of these states is also difficult to assess. Both Vietnam and Laos have been deeply affected by the collapse of their former patron, the Soviet Union. Vietnam managed to start *Do Moi*, the new policy of agricultural and economic reform, before the end of Soviet aid. This allowed them to survive economically, even to prosper, but it also delayed the need for the political reforms that have swept the other states in the Soviet circle (except Cuba). The Vietnamese domination of Laos continues, and the Lao Politburo shows no sign, yet, of any eagerness for reform. But Laos is caught in a different dynamic from Vietnam, or from most other countries in the former Soviet sphere; it has a heroin economy, and its fate is thus linked to another axis: Burma, China, and the cartels that control this hugely lucrative industry. Drug economies are by their very nature anti-democratic. They require secrecy, closed banking systems and special borders, they reward only corruption, and they are invariably controlled by armed and violent elites. Laos's future, like that of the Shan and Wa nationalities in Burma, depends to a considerable degree on the fate of the drug trade, a reality that will not be easily resolved in either case. Drug cartels do not want empowered populations any more than juntas do.

Malaysia and Thailand are arguably the 'most likely to succeed' of the countries discussed. The educational levels of their populations and the complexity of their economies bode well for movements toward greater democracy, accountability, and improvements in health and education. But these are not large countries and they cannot exist in isolation from their neighbors. As long as HIV and heroin, to take only the examples we have focused on, continue to rage out of control in Burma, Thailand's successes will be under constant threat. With the immensity of Indonesia at its door, Malaysia too must tread carefully to avoid authoritarian leanings. This is a dynamic region and change has been swift and continuous for almost two decades. It is likely to continue. The changes could lead to increased prosperity, stability, and peace, or in other directions. The more the people of these countries have a say in shaping this future, the more likely it will be that their aspirations for health, education, and justice will be fulfilled. In the words of Maha Ghosananda, one step at a time.

Will HIV affect these dynamic trends? And if so, how?

Empowerment for the women of Southeast Asia is clearly going to be a cornerstone of democratic developments in the region. Indeed, it is striking how many of the region's progressive leaders – Corazon Aquino, Aung San Suu Kyi, Megawati Sukarnoputri – have been women. But while slavery continues to exist, and women from the poorest and most chaotic social settings continue to be trafficked and sold, women's empowerment is likely to be delayed. There has not been a great deal of solidarity between feminists and sex workers in Southeast Asia, apart from groups like EMPOWER, but this solidarity, I would argue, is an essential step on the path to equality and respect for all the region's women, and thus for democracy. The model for this kind of bridge building does exist, and comes from an unexpected source: Cambodia. Cambodian women have suffered hugely in the last 50 years, and are only just beginning to organize and to play political roles in the difficult rebirth of the state. But the feminist movement there, embodied in the Cambodia Women's Development Association (CWDA), has explicitly linked the sex trade to the larger issue of the treatment of women, the poor, and human rights. They have taken the government to task, supported sex workers in the courts, challenged the policies of the police, and worked with foreign NGOs to protect trafficked children in the sex trade. This is a fragile movement in a country where fire-power rules, but it is in this kind of coming together that hope for HIV/AIDS control lies. If the empowerment of some women fails to address the women in the sex industry, it will have little effect on the AIDS crisis. And if men continue to feel comfortable paying for sex with slaves, their wives may achieve little in the direction of true empowerment.

The motto of the CWDA is: There is no sustainable development where violence and the commodification of women exits.

Note

1. Burma and Laos were admitted as ASEAN's eighth and ninth member states in June 1997. Cambodia's entry was delayed owing to the *coup d'état* of Hun Sen.

22. Conclusion: condoms or land-mines

My humble opinion is that without the commitment of leadership at the highest level to preventing further spread of AIDS, we will never see the scale of action necessary to address this issue and its social and economic consequences.

AIDS must be viewed as a national development issue. If we present AIDS as a health problem, it will be treated as such. AIDS is not a health problem, it is a behavioral and societal problem – and an urgent national development priority. Today, AIDS remains the most critical threat to the social and economic progress of the region [Asia and the Pacific] – along with environmental degradation.

The leaders of our countries are not taking AIDS seriously enough. I am here today to tell you about my view as the former Prime Minister of a country facing one of the fastest-spreading AIDS epidemics on the planet, in the hope that we can get more leaders to take AIDS more seriously. We need more action!

Anand Panyarachun, former Prime Minister of Thailand, addressing the Third International Conference on AIDS in Asia and the Pacific, 21 September 1995, Chiang Mai, Thailand.

Prevention works. HIV-prevention is possible, even in resource-limited settings. Accountable governments and active public programs can reduce the burden of AIDS and reduce unnecessary suffering. Civil strife, repression, human rights abuses, censorship, corruption, and government neglect can make HIV epidemics worse. Government inaction can add the grief and losses of AIDS to people already burdened. The choice for governments, as a Canadian social theorist put it, is between condoms and land-mines, investments in life or in death, improved health or increased suffering.

Morality aside, investments in disease prevention and health promotion are also investments in development, as Khun Anand's eloquent speech attests. Investments in land-mines may preserve power elites, may prolong the political lives of parties or individuals, but they can never lead to development. They only add to suffering.

Countries ultimately have to choose which way they will go, but governments should be held accountable for those choices. Governments and ideologies which by their actions decrease the health of peoples, or fail to sustain it, are failures, as are those that fail to prepare the young for adult life, and those regimes that degrade the sanctity of ordinary human beings. By these criteria there are some glaring political failures in Southeast Asia. It is only logical that theirs should be the countries most affected by HIV. Near the end of the speech excerpted above, Khun Anand suggested that Asian Development Bank support for development should be linked to a country's commitment to HIV prevention. Spending money on condoms would lead to more money for development. This is the kind of approach that could save millions of lives, and could lead to support for real development, which implies empowerment, participation, and liberation, and to real health, which is more than a state of personal well-being: it is a people's achievement, created and sustained by a just society. It is physical, emotional, and *shared*.

Suffering also is shared. Burma and Cambodia have shown us that the spread of HIV is aided and abetted by social chaos. The four horsemen come at once, not separately.

We can do better. We have the tools now. There is no magic bullet for HIV, but there are few magic bullets for anything. What we need are candid, funded, culture-specific prevention programs. This will still be true if, and when, an HIV vaccine is available. Polio vaccine is cheap and available, yet polio continues to kill and cripple children in many of the countries now struggling with HIV.

The choices are clear. We need more action. Wars in the blood can be won.

Bibliography

1. Introduction

Agence France Press, 'AIDS looms as threat to Asian Economic boom', *Bangkok Post*, Wednesday, August 3, 1994.

AIDSCAP, UNAIDS, Harvard School of Public Health, 'The Status and Trends of the Global HIV/AIDS Pandemic', *11th International Conference on AIDS, Vancouver, Satellite Symposium Final Report*, July 1996.

Bond, K.C., D.D. Celentano, Phonsophakul and C. Vaddhanaphuti, 'Mobility and Migration: Female Commercial Sex Work and the HIV epidemic in Northern Thailand', in G. Herdt (ed.), *Sexual Cultures and Migration in the Era of AIDS: Anthropological and Demographic Perspectives*, Oxford University Press, New York, 1998.

Brookmeyer, R. and M. Gail, *AIDS Epidemiology: a quantitative approach*, Oxford University Press, New York, 1994.

Brummelhuis, H.T. and G. Herdt (eds.), *Culture and Sexual Risk: Anthropologic Perspectives on AIDS*, Gordon & Breach, Amsterdam, 1996.

Cartwright, F., *Disease and History*, Dorset Press, New York, 1972.

Chin, J., 'Scenarios for the AIDS epidemic in Asia', *Asia–Pacific Population Research Reports*, Vol. 1, No. 2, 1995.

Mann, J., D. Tarantola and T. Netter, *AIDS in the World*, Harvard University Press, Cambridge, Mass., 1992.

Nelson, K.E., D.D. Celentano, S. Eiumtrakul, D.R. Hoover, C. Beyrer, S. Suprasert, S. Kuntolbutra and C. Khamboonruang, 'Changes in sexual behavior and a decline in HIV infection among young men in Thailand', *New England Journal of Medicine*, Vol. 335, 1996, pp. 279–303.

Osborne, M., *Southeast Asia: An Introduction* (6th edn), Silkworm Books, Bangkok, 1996.

Panyarachun, A., Address to the Third International Conference on AIDS in Asia and the Pacific, Chiang Mai, Thailand, September 21, 1995. An excerpt from this speech can be found on p. 222.

Royal Thai Ministry of Public Health, Division of Communicable Disease Control Region 10, HIV Sentinel Surveillance, 1995, Bangkok.

Sittitrai, W., P. Phanuphak, J. Barry and T. Brown, 'Thai Sexual Behavior and Risk of HIV infection: A Report of the 1990 Survey of Partner Relations and Risk of HIV Infection in Thailand', Thai Red Cross Society and Chulalongkorn University Press, Bangkok, 1992.

Viravaidya, M., S.A. Obremsky and C. Myers, 'The Economic Impact of AIDS on Thailand', in *The Economic Implications of AIDS in Asia*, UNDP Publications, New Delhi, 1993.

Way, P.O. and K. Stanecki, 'The demographic impact of an AIDS epidemic on an African country: Application of the IWGAIDS model', Center for International Research, Staff paper 58, US Bureau of the Census, Washington D.C., 1991.
Zinsser, H., *Rats, Lice and History*, Little, Brown, Boston, 1934.

2. Thailand

Beyrer, C., 'The Kingdom of Lanna and the HIV Epidemic', *The Journal of The Siam Society*, Vol. 83, Parts 1&2, 1995, pp. 221–30.
Celentano, D., K. Nelson, S. Suprasert et al., 'Behavioral and Socio-Demographic Risks for Frequent Visits to Commercial Sex Workers among Northern Thai Men', *AIDS*, Vol. 7, 1993, pp. 1646–52.
Coedes, G., *The Indianized States of Southeast Asia*, University of Hawaii Press, Honolulu, 1973.
Ekachai, S., Presentation at 'Women and AIDS in Thailand' Symposium, Chiang Mai, 1993.
Hanenberg, R., W. Rojanapithayakorn, P. Kunasol and D. Sokal, 'Impact of Thailand's HIV-control programme as indicated by the decline of sexually transmitted diseases', *The Lancet*, Vol. 344, 1994, pp. 243–5.
Kitayaporn, D., S. Tansuphaswadikul, P. Lohsomboon et al., 'Survival of AIDS Patients in the Emerging Epidemic in Bangkok, Thailand', *Journal of AIDS & Human Retrovirology*, Vol. 11, 1996, pp. 77–82.
Kunanusont, C., H.M. Foy, J.K. Kreiss et al., 'HIV-1 subtypes and male-to-female transmission in Thailand', *The Lancet*, Vol. 345, 1995, pp. 1078–83.
Kunawararak, P., C. Beyrer, C. Natpratan et al., 'The epidemiology of HIV and syphilis among male commercial sex workers in northern Thailand', *AIDS*, Vol. 9, 1995, pp. 171–6.
Limonanda, B., 'Female Commercial Sex Workers and AIDS: Perspectives from Thai Rural Communities', 5th International Conference on Thai Studies, University of London, 1993.
Mastro, T.M. and K. Limpakarnjanarat, 'Condom use in Thailand: how much is it slowing the HIV/AIDS epidemic?', *AIDS*, Vol. 9, 1995, pp. 523–5.
McCutchan, F., 'HIV Genetic Diversity', plenary address at the 9th International Conference on AIDS, Vancouver, 1996.
Muecke, M., 'Mother Sold Food, Daughter Sells Her Body: The Cultural Continuity of Prostitution', *Social Science and Medicine*, Vol. 35, 1992, pp. 891–6.
Nelson, K., D. Celentano, S. Suprasert et al., 'Risk Factors for HIV Infection Among Young Adult Men in Northern Thailand', *JAMA*, Vol. 270, 1993, pp. 955–60.
Nelson, K.E., V. Suriyanon, E. Taylor et al., 'The incidence of HIV-1 infections in village populations of northern Thailand,' *AIDS*, Vol. 8, 1994, pp. 951–5.
Nopkesorn, T., T. Mastro, S. Sangkharomya, M. Sweat, P. Singharaj, K. Limpakarnjanarat, H. Gayle and B. Weniger, 'HIV-1 Infection in Young Men in Northern Thailand', *AIDS*, Vol. 7, 1993, pp. 1233–9.
Ou, C-Y., Y. Takebe, C-C. Lou et al., 'Wide Distribution of Two Subtypes of HIV-1 in Thailand', *AIDS Research and Human Retroviruses*, Vol. 8, 1992, pp. 1471–2.

Reynolds, C.J. (ed.), *National Identity and its Defenders: Thailand 1939–1989*, Silkworm Books, Bangkok, 1991.

Royal Thai Ministry of Public Health, Division of Communicable Disease Control HIV/AIDS Surveillance Data, Bangkok, 1995.

Sawanpanyalert, P., K. Ungshusak, S. Thanprasertsuk and P. Akarasewi, 'HIV-1 seroconversion rates among female commercial sex workers, Chiang Mai, Thailand: a multi cross-sectional study', *AIDS*, Vol. 8, 1994, pp. 825–9.

Siraprapasiri, J., S. Thanprasertsuk, A. Rodklay, S. Srivanichakorn, P. Sawanpanyalert and J. Temtanarak, 'Risk Factors for HIV Among Prostitutes in Chiang Mai, Thailand', *AIDS*, Vol. 5, 1991, pp. 579–82.

Ungphakorn, J., W. Sittitrai, 'The Thai response to the HIV/AIDS epidemic', *AIDS*, Vol. 8 (suppl. 2), 1994, pp. S155–63.

Weniger, B.G., K. Limpakarnjanarat, K. Ungchusak et al., 'The epidemiology of HIV infection and AIDS in Thailand', *AIDS*, Vol. 5 (suppl. 2), 1991. pp. S71–85.

Weniger, B.G., Y. Takebe, C-Y. Ou and S. Yamazaki, 'The Molecular Epidemiology of HIV in Asia', *AIDS*, Vol. 8 (suppl. 2), 1994.

Wright, J.J., *The Balancing Act*, Asia Books, Bangkok, 1991.

Wyatt, D.K., *Thailand: A short history*, Yale University Press, New Haven, 1984.

3. Burma

Aung San Suu Kyi, *Freedom from Fear*, Penguin Books, London, 1991.

Amnesty International, 'Myanmar: Conditions in Prisons and Labour Camps', *ASA* 16/22/95, London, 1995.

Boston Globe, editorial, 'Burma's heroin deal', Boston, November 27, 1996.

Boucaud, A. and L. Boucaud, *Burma's Golden Triangle*, Asia Books, Bangkok, 1992.

Brown, T., 'HIV and AIDS in Asia: Japan Conference Review', *AIDS Care*, Vol. 7, No. 1, 1995, pp. 71–6.

Department of Health, Yangon, 'Annual Report of the AIDS Prevention and Control Programme, Myanmar 1994', Disease Control Programme, Yangon, 1995.

Federation of Trade Unions–Burma, 'Government Hospital Staff Conditions in Burma', presentation at the First HIV/AIDS Policy Forum on Burma, 1996.

Htoon, M.T., San Lwin and Thwe Zan, 'HIV/AIDS Situation in Myanmar', *AIDS*, Vol. 8 (suppl. 2), 1994.

Human Rights Watch/Asia, 'Human Rights in Burma in 1991', Vol. 4, No. 24, 1992.

Isett, S., 'Burma's Victims of Apathy', *Bangkok Post*, September 16, 1994, p. 36.

Lintner, B., *Burma in Revolt: Opium and Insurgency since 1948*, White Lotus, Bangkok, 1995.

Lintner, B., *Outrage*, White Lotus, Bangkok, 1994.

National Coalition Government of the Union of Burma, *Burma: Human Rights Yearbook, 1995*, NCGUB Press, Bangkok, 1995.

Reuters, 'Khun Sa thrives after rebuilding empire', *Bangkok Post*, January 4, 1997, p. A2.

Soe, Win Zaw et al., 'Some Characteristics of Hospitalized HIV Seropositive Patients in Myanmar', *Southeast Asian Journal of Tropical Medicine & Public Health*,

Vol. 24, No. 1, 1993.

Southeast Asian Information Network, *Out of Control; the HIV/AIDS Epidemic in Burma*, SAIN, Chiang Mai, 1995.

Smith, M., *Burma: Insurgency and the Politics of Ethnicity*, Zed Books Ltd, London, 1993.

Smith, M., *Fatal Silence: Freedom of Expression and the Right to Health in Burma*, Article 19, London, 1996.

Stimson, G., 'HIV Infection and Injecting Drug Use in the Union of Myanmar', United Nations International Drug Control Programme, Vienna, 1994.

Thaung, B., K.M. Gyee and B. Kywe, 'Rapid Assessment study of Drug Abuse in Myanmar: A Ministry of Health & UNDCP Co-Sponsored Project', 9th International Conference on AIDS, Vancouver, Abstract Tu.C.2547, 1996.

Ti, T., H. Naing, P. Noe, H. Yanai and K. Nakamoto, 'HIV Seroprevalence study in patients attending Union Tuberculosis Institute, Yangon (1994, November and December)', Third International Conference on AIDS in Asia and the Pacific, Chiang Mai, Abstract PB128, 1995.

Unicef, 'Possibilities for a United Nations Peace and Development Initiative for Myanmar', Unpublished Draft for Consultation, Rangoon, 1992.

Yokota, Y., 'Report on the situation of human rights in Myanmar, prepared by the Special Rapporteur, Mr. Yozo Yokota, in accordance with Commission resolution 1995/72', United Nations, Geneva, 1996. The reply of the junta to Yokota's charges also makes interesting reading: 'State Law and Order Restoration Council response to the report of the Special Rapporteur, Mr. Yozo Yokota, in accordance with Commission resolution 1995/72', United Nations, Geneva, 1996.

4. Cambodia

Anon., 'AIDS a bigger danger to army than Khmer Rouge', *Bangkok Post*, July 17, 1995, p. A3.

Anon., 'AIDS threatens future of Cambodia's military', *The Nation*, Bangkok, July 18, 1996, p. 1.

Anon., 'Cambodia returnees bring home HIV', *AIDS Weekly*, India, September 20, 1993, pp. 12–13.

Artenstein, A.W., J. Coppola, A.E. Brown, J.K. Carr et al., 'Multiple introductions of HIV-1 subtype E into the Western Hemisphere', *The Lancet*, Vol. 346, 1995, pp. 1198–9.

Beyrer, C., 'Burma and Cambodia: Human Rights, Social Disruption, and the Spread of HIV/AIDS', *Health and Human Rights*, 1997.

Brodine, S.K., J.R. Mascola, P.J. Weiss et al., 'Detection of diverse HIV-1 subtypes in the United States', *The Lancet*, Vol. 346, 1995, pp. 1199–1200.

Bedford, M., 'Cambodia – Still Waiting for Peace', in *Indochina Interchange*, Oxfam, Boston, 1995.

Cambodian Human Rights Foundation, 'Rapid Appraisal of the Human Rights Vigilance of Cambodia on Child Prostitution and Trafficking, March–April 1995', CHRF, Phnom Penh, 1995.

Cambodian Women's Development Association, 'Prostitution and Traffic of Women: A Dialogue on the Cambodian Situation', CWDA Special Reports, Phnom Penh, 1996.

Chandler, D.P., *A History of Cambodia* (2nd edition), Westview, Boulder, 1993.
Chang, P.M., *Kampuchea Between China and Vietnam*, Singapore University Press, Singapore, 1987.
Chanthou, B., 'Grim picture of women's lot', *Phnom Penh Post*, Phnom Penh, June 1, 1995.
Escoffier, C., 'Sexually transmitted diseases in Banteay Meanchey [Cambodia]', Médecins Sans Frontières, 1995.
Ghosananda, M., *Step by Step*, Parallax Press, Berkeley, 1992.
Kongkea, R., 'AIDS victims on the rise', *Phnom Penh Post*, Phnom Penh, April 3, 1996.
Land-Mines Advisory Group, Information on the land mine situation in Cambodia was kindly provided to the author by staff of the Land-Mines Advisory Group, Phnom Penh, 1996.
Reuters, 'Cambodian editor wounded in shooting', *Bangkok Post*, January 4, 1997, p. A2. Lang Samnang, 26, and editor of the independent *Idea for Cambodia's Children* was shot after months of threats and warnings from the CPP. Three other journalists have been murdered in Cambodia since 1994.
Reuters, 'Japanese troops get AIDS virus in Cambodia', *Sankei Shimbun*, Tokyo, October 20, 1993, p. 1.
Saddhatissa, H. (ed.), *Sutta Nipata*, Salem House, Cambridge, 1985.
Sherry, A., M. Lee, M. Vatikiotis, 'For Lust or Money', *Far Eastern Economic Review*, Hong Kong, Vol. 3, 1995.
Tia, P. et al., 'The Epidemiology of HIV in Cambodia', Tenth International Conference on AIDS, Yokohama, abstract PC0621, 1994.

5. Laos

Chan, S. (ed.), *Hmong Means Free*, Temple University Press, Philadelphia, 1994.
Dommen, A.J., *Laos: Keystone of Indochina*, Westview Press, London, 1985.
Finch, P. and S. Chantavanich (eds.), 'The Lao Returnees in the Voluntary Repatriation Programme from Thailand', *Indochina Chronology*, Occasional Papers Series No. 03, Indochinese Refugee Information Center, January–March, 1995.
Gunn, C.G., *Rebellion in Laos: peasant and politics in a colonial backwater*, Westview Press, Boulder, 1990.
Hamilton-Merritt, J., *Tragic Mountains: The Hmong, The Americans, and the Secret Wars for Laos, 1942–1992*, Indiana University Press, Indianapolis, 1993.
Lintner, B., *Outrage*, White Lotus, Bangkok, 1994.
Lintner, B., *Burma: Opium and Insurgency since 1948*, White Lotus, Bangkok, 1995.
Prasongsith, B.C., P. Blanche, K. Phouvang et al., 'HIV Infection in Lao Republic', 10th International Conference on AIDS, Yokohama, 1994.
McCoy, A.W., *The Politics of Heroin in Southeast Asia*, HarperCollins, New York, 1972.

6. Malaysia

Asia Watch, *A Modern Form of Slavery, Trafficking of Burmese Women and Girls into Brothels in Thailand*, Asia Watch/Human Rights Watch, Bangkok, 1993.
Anti-Narcotics Task Force, Malaysia, 'Malaysia Narcotics Report 1994', National Security Council, Prime Minister's Department, Kuala Lumpur, 1994.

Beyrer, C., K.P. Ng, T. Van Cott et al., 'HIV-1 subtypes in Malaysia determined serologically', submitted to *AIDS & Human Retroviruses*, 1997.

Brown, T.M., K.E. Robbins, M. Sinniah et al., 'HIV Type 1 Subtypes in Malaysia Include B, C, and E', *AIDS & Human Retroviruses*, Vol. 12, 1996, pp. 1655–7.

East–West Center, 'AIDS in Asia: the gathering storm', University of Hawaii, Honolulu, 1994.

Lam, S.K., 'HIV and AIDS – The Road Ahead', proceedings of Workshop on the Epidemiology of HIV and AIDS, Kuala Lumpur, 1996.

Limonanda, B., 'Demographic and Behavioral Study of Female Commercial Sex Workers in Thailand', Special Report, Institute of Population Studies, Chulalongkorn University, Bangkok, 1993.

Limonanda, B., G.S.D. van Griensven, N. Changvatana et al., 'Condom use and risk factors for HIV-1 infection among female commercial sex workers in Thailand', *American Journal of Public Health*, Vol. 84, 1994, pp. 2026–7.

Ministry of Health, Malaysia, *Reporting of HIV/AIDS in Malaysia*, AIDS/STD Section, Kuala Lumpur, 1996.

Royal Thai Ministry of Public Health, Division of Communicable Disease Control, HIV/AIDS Surveillance Data, Bangkok, 1995.

Singh, J. et al., *AIDS*, Vol. 8 (suppl. 2), 1994, pp. 99–103.

Sittitrai, W., *The Sun*, Kuala Lumpur, Malaysia, July 19, 1995, p. 8.

Tsuchide, H., T.S. Saraswathy, M. Sinniah et al., 'HIV-1 variants in South and South-East Asia', *International Journal of STD & AIDS*, Vol. 6, 1995, pp. 117–220.

7. Vietnam

CARE International Vietnam, 'Targeting Young Men: AIDS Prevention in Vietnam', Special Report, CARE, Hanoi, 1994.

CARE International Vietnam, 'An Audience Analysis of Urban Men and Sex Workers', Special Report, CARE, Hanoi, 1993.

Franklin, B., I. Brugemann, 'Women and the risk of HIV/AIDS in Vietnam', *AIDS Analysis Asia*, Vol. 4, 1995.

Franklin, B. and N.T. Khanh, 'The Fire in the Dragon: A Study of Risk Factors for HIV/AIDS Among Urban Men and Commercial Sex Workers in Vietnam', 10th International Conference on AIDS, Yokohama, Abstract 031D, 1984.

Huong, N.D., 'Tuberculosis and HIV Infection in Vietnam', Third International Conference on AIDS in Asia and the Pacific, Chiang Mai, Abstract PB127, 1995.

Kahane, T., 'Turning the Tide', *Asia Week*, April 10, 1996.

Ministry of Health, Vietnam, Report of the National AIDS Control Committee, Hanoi, 1995.

Nguyen, N.N.T. and T.O. Nguyen, *Will to Live: An oral history of five people who are found to be HIV-Positive*, CARE International in Vietnam, Hanoi, 1995.

Sheehan, N., *Two Cities: Hanoi and Saigon*, Jonathan Cape, London, 1992.

UNAIDS, 'The Status and Trends of the Global HIV/AIDS Pandemic', 11th International Conference on AIDS, Vancouver, Satellite Symposium Final Report, Geneva, 1996.

8. Yunnan

Chin, J., 'Scenarios for the AIDS epidemic in Asia', *Asia–Pacific Population Research Reports*, No. 2, 1995.

Chuang, C-Y., P-Y. Chang and K-C. Lin, 'AIDS in the Republic of China', *Clinical Infectious Diseases*,Vol. 17 (suppl. 2), 1993, pp. S337–40.

Cowley, G., 'China: When AIDS Finally Hits', in *Newsweek*, April 15, 1996.

Department of Disease Control, Ministry of Health, *AIDS Prevention and Control in China*, China Pictorial Publishing House, Beijing, 1994.

Ji, Y., F. Tang, Z. Ji et al., 'Exploration of Treatment of AIDS with Living Toads', presentation at the International Symposium on AIDS, Beijing, China, 1995.

Lintner, B., *Burma in Revolt: Opium and Insurgency since 1948*, White Lotus, Bangkok, 1995, contains some fascinating historical information on the origins of the modern drug routes in the region.

Spartacus, *Spartacus International Gay Guide*, Bruno Gmunder, Berlin, 1995–96.

Tyler, P.E., 'Heroin Influx Ignites a Growing AIDS Epidemic in China', *New York Times*, November 28, 1995.

Yu, E.S.H., X. Qiyi, Z. Konglai et al., 'HIV Infection and AIDS in China, 1985–1994', *American Journal of Public Health*, Vol. 86, 1996, pp. 1116–22.

Zeng Yi, 'The Working Situation of Controlling and Preventing AIDS in China', presentation at The International Symposium on AIDS, Beijing, China, 1995.

Zunyou Wu, R. Detels, Jiangpeng Zhang et al., 'Risk Factors for Intravenous Drug Use and Sharing of Equipment Among Young Male Drug Users in Southwest China', presentation at The International Symposium on AIDS, Beijing, China, 1995.

9. Women

Anon., 'Bringing AZT to Poor Countries', *Science*, Vol. 269, No. 4, 1995, pp. 624–5.

Burton, R. (trans.), in A.H. Walton (ed.), *The Perfumed Garden of the Shaykh Nefzawi*, Gramercy Publishing Co., New York, 1964.

Brown, T., W. Sittitrai, S. Vanichseni et al., 'The recent epidemiology of HIV and AIDS in Thailand', *AIDS*, Vol. 8 (suppl. 2), 1994, pp. S131–41.

Connor, E.M., R.S. Sperling, R. Gelbert et al., 'Reduction of maternal–infant transmission of human immunodeficiency virus type 1 with zidovudine treatment', *New England Journal of Medicine*, Vol. 331, 1994, pp. 1173–80.

Elias, C., 'Sexually Transmitted Diseases and the Reproductive Health of Women in Developing Countries', The Population Council, Working Paper 5, 1991.

Fleming, P.S., 'Access to Treatments in Developing Countries', address at the 11th International Conference on AIDS, Vancouver, 1996.

Nelson, K.E., D.D. Celentano, S. Eiumtrakul, D.R. Hoover, C. Beyrer et al., 'Changes in sexual behavior and a decline in HIV infection among young men in Thailand', *New England Journal of Medicine*, Vol. 335, 1996, pp. 279–303.

Wasserheit, J., 'Epidemiologic Synergy: Interrelationships between Human Immunodeficiency Virus Infection and Other Sexually Transmitted Diseases', *Sexually Transmitted Diseases*, Vol. 19, 1991, pp. 62–4.

For a thorough discussion of heterosexual transmission of HIV, see also I. De

Vincenzi (for the European Study Group on Heterosexual Transmission of HIV), 'A longitudinal study of human immunodeficiency virus transmission by heterosexual partners', *New England Journal of Medicine*, Vol. 331, 1994, pp. 341–6.

10. The Flesh Trade

Albert, A.E., D.L. Warner, R.A. Hatcher, J. Trussel and C. Bennett, 'Condom Use among Female Commercial Sex Workers in Nevada's Legal Brothels', *American Journal of Public Health*, Vol. 85, 1995, pp. 1514–20.

Cambodian Women's Development Association, Mission Statement, 1995.

Cambodian Women's Development Association, 'Prostitution and Traffic of Women and Children', conference report, Phnom Penh, 1995.

Downs, A.M., I. De Vincenzi, 'Probability of Heterosexual Transmission of HIV: Relationship to the Number of Unprotected Sexual Contacts', *Journal of AIDS and Human Retrovirology*, Vol. 11, 1996, pp. 388–95.

Estebanez, P., K. Fitch, R. Najera, 'HIV and female sex workers', *Bulletin of the World Health Organization*, Vol. 71, No. 3/4, 1993, pp. 397–412.

Fairclough, G, 'Doing the Dirty Work: Asia's brothels thrive on migrant labour', *Far Eastern Economic Review*, December 14, 1995. pp. 27–28.

Federation of Trade Unions–Burma, 'A survey of the HIV/AIDS & Migrant Workers Situation in Ranong', *FTUB Special Report*, Washington, D.C., 1996.

Holthausen, J., 'Burma's AIDS Crisis', *Het Parool*, December 1, 1996, p. A1 (in Dutch).

Hunt, C., 'Migrant labor and sexually transmitted disease: AIDS in Africa', *Journal of Health and Human Behavior*, Vol. 30, 1989, pp. 353–73.

Institute of Population Studies, Chulalongkorn University, 'Surveys of Commercial Sex Workers in Sugai Kolok, Narathiwat Province and Batong, Yala Province, 1994', presentation at the Consultation on Information and Population Movement and HIV/AIDS, Bangkok, Thailand, 1996.

Mastro, T.M., G.A. Satten, T. Nopkesorn, S. Sangkharomya and I.M. Longini, 'Probability of female-to-male transmission of HIV-1 in Thailand', *The Lancet*, Vol. 343, 1994, pp. 204–7.

McKeganey, N.P., 'Prostitution and HIV: what do we know and where might research be targeted in the future?', *AIDS*, Vol. 8, 1994, pp. 1215–26.

Plummer, F.A., K. Fowke, N.J.D. Nagelkerke et al., 'Resistance to HIV among continuously exposed prostitutes in Nairobi', 11th International Conference on AIDS, Berlin, Abstract WS-AO7-3, 1993.

Pollock, J., 'Migrant Workers and Discrimination', address at the First Policy Forum on Addressing the AIDS Epidemic in Burma, 1996.

Pramaulratana, A., presentation at the First Technical Consultation on Migration and AIDS, Asian Institute of Population Studies, Chulalongkorn University, Bangkok, 1995.

Reade, R., G. Richwald and N. Williams, 'The Nevada legal brothel system as a model for AIDS prevention among female sex industry workers', Sixth International Conference on AIDS, San Francisco, 1990.

Royal Thai Ministry of the Interior, quoted by G. Risser, 'Population Movements in South-East Asia', Asian Research Center for Migration, Chulalongkorn University, Bangkok, 1994.

Rowland-Jones, S., J. Sutton, K. Ariyoshi et al., 'HIV-specific cytotoxic T-cells in HIV-exposed but uninfected Gambian women', *Nature Medicine*, Vol. 1, 1995, pp. 59–64.

Royal Thai Ministry of the Interior, Thai National Labor Statistics, Bangkok, 1995.

Shrey, A., M. Lee and M. Vatiklotis, 'Sex Trade; For Lust or Money', *Far Eastern Economic Review*, December 14, 1995, pp. 22–3.

United Nations High Commission for Refugees, 'Response to CWDA allegations of UNTAC's role in trafficking in Cambodia', Phnom Penh Conference on Traffic of Women and Children, 1995.

Vanaspong, C., 'Prostitution: New Law Won't Help', *Bangkok Post*, April 7, 1996, p. 17.

11. Military Studies

Anon., 'The Profits and Losses of AIDS', *The Economist*, July 13, 1996, pp. 81–2.

Anon., 'AIDS threatens future of Cambodia's military', *The Nation*, Bangkok, July 18, 1996, p. 1.

Altman, L.K., 'After Setback, First Large AIDS Vaccine Trials are Planned', *New York Times*, November 29, 1994, pp. B6–7.

Levin, L.I., T.A. Peterman, P.O. Renzullo et al., 'HIV-1 Seroconversion and Risk Behaviors among Young Men in the US Army', *American Journal of Public Health*, Vol. 85, 1995, pp. 1500–1506.

Nelson, K.E., D.D. Celentano, S. Suprasert et al., 'Risk factors for HIV infection among young adult men in northern Thailand', *JAMA*, Vol. 270, No. 8, 1993.

Nelson, K.E., D.D. Celentano, S. Eiumtrakul et al., 'Changes in sexual behavior and a decline in HIV infection among young men in Thailand', *New England Journal of Medicine*, Vol. 335, 1996, pp. 297–303.

Shilts, R., *Conduct Unbecoming: Gays & Lesbians in the U.S. Military*, St. Martins Press, New York, 1993.

Thein, M.T., S. Than, B. Kywe et al., 'Sexual Risk Behaviors in Young Soldiers' HIV & VDRL Seroprevalence', Dept. of Defense Medical Services, Myanmar, 3rd International Conference on AIDS in Asia and the Pacific, Chiang Mai, Thailand, Abstract B304, 1995.

Verghese, B.G., *India's Resurgent Northeast: Ethnicity, Insurgency, Governance, Development*, Center for Policy Research, Konark, Delhi, 1996.

12. Chasing the Dragon

Celentano, D.D., A. Munoz, S. Cohn, K.E. Nelson and D. Vlahov, 'Drug-related behavior change for HIV transmission among injection drug users', *Addiction*, Vol. 89, 1994, pp. 1309–17.

Choopanya, K., S. Vanichseni, D.C. Des Jarlais et al., 'Risk factors and HIV seropositivity among injecting drug users in Bangkok', *International Journal of Addictions*, Vol. 26, 1991, pp. 1333–47.

Des Jarlais, D.C., M. Marmor, D. Paono et al., 'HIV incidence among injecting drug users in New York City syringe exchange programmes', *The Lancet*, Vol. 348, 1996, pp. 987–91.

Merson, M., 'Returning Home: reflections on the USA's response to the HIV/AIDS epidemic', in *The Lancet*, Vol. 347, 1996, pp. 1673–6. This presents a lucid analysis of US prevention policy and its limitations.

Nelson, K.E., 'The epidemiology of HIV infection among injecting drug users and other risk populations in Thailand', *AIDS*, Vol. 8, 1994, pp. 1499–1500.

Nelson, K.E., D. Vlahov, S. Cohn et al., 'Human Immunodeficiency Virus Infection in Diabetic Intravenous Drug Users', *JAMA*, Vol. 266, 1991, pp. 2259–61.

Phanupak, P., V. Posyachinda, T. Uenklabh and W. Rojanapithayakorn, 'HIV transmission among intravenous drug abusers', 5th International Conference on AIDS, Montreal, Abstract TG025, 1989.

Shilts, R., *And the Band Played On: Politics, People, and the AIDS Epidemic*, St. Martin's Press, New York, 1987.

Vanichseni, S., B. Wongsuwan, K. Choopanya and K. Wongpanich, 'A controlled trial of methadone maintenance in a population of intravenous drug users in Bangkok: implications for prevention of HIV', *International Journal of Addictions*, Vol. 26, 1991, pp. 1313–20.

Weniger, B. and T. Brown, 'The March of AIDS Through Asia', *New England Journal of Medicine*, Vol. 335, No. 5, 1995, pp. 343–4.

Xia, M., J.K. Kreiss and K.K. Holmes, 'Risk Factors for HIV infection among drug users in Yunnan Province, China: association with intravenous drug use and protective effect of boiling reusable needles and syringes', 9th International Conference on AIDS, Berlin, Abstract WS-C15-1, 1993.

13. Tribes

Beyrer, C., S. Suprasert, W. Sittitrai et al., 'Widely varying prevalence and risk behaviors and HIV infection among the Hilltribe and ethnic minority peoples of upper northern Thailand', *AIDS Care*, 1997.

Filbeck, D., 'The Lua of Nan Province', *Journal of the Siam Society*, Vol. 77, Part 1, 1989, pp. 102–9.

Gray, J., 'The social and sexual mobility of young women in rural northern Thailand – Khon Muang and Hilltribes', paper presented at the First Workshop on Sociocultural Dimensions of HIV/AIDS Control and Care in Thailand, Chiang Mai, 1994.

Hamilton, J.W., *Pwo Karen: At the edge of mountain and plain*, West Publ. Co., St. Paul, 1976.

Kammerer, C. et al., 'Vulnerability to HIV Infection Among Three Hill Tribes in Northern Thailand', in H.T. Brummelhuis and G. Herdt (eds.), *Culture and Sexual Risk: Anthropologic Perspectives on AIDS*, Gordon & Breach, Amsterdam, 1996.

Kammerer, C., O. Klein Hutheesing, R. Maneeprasert and P. Symonds, 'Vulnerability to HIV infection among three hill tribes in northern Thailand: Qualitative anthropological issues', presentation at the 5th International Conference on Thai Studies, SOAS, London, 1993.

Klein Hutheesing, O., 'Linking the Lisu to the HIV/AIDS Epidemic: Observations of a Cultural-Political Kind', paper presented at the First Workshop on Sociocultural Dimensions of HIV/AIDS Control and Care in Thailand, Chiang Mai, 1994.

Kunstadter, P., 'Cultural factors related to transmission and control of HIV infection: Highland minorities of northern Thailand', paper presented at the First Workshop on Sociocultural Dimensions of HIV/AIDS Control and Care in Thailand, Chiang Mai, 1994.

Lewis, P. and E. Lewis, *Peoples of the Golden Triangle*, Thames and Hudson, London, 1984.

Milne, L., *The Shans at Home*, Paragon Books, New York, 1970.

Symonds, P., 'The Political and Cultural Economy of the Hmong as related to HIV/AIDS: Observations from the field', paper presented at the First Workshop on Sociocultural Dimensions of HIV/AIDS Control and Care in Thailand, Chiang Mai, 1994.

Thai National Statistics Office, *Summary Report of the Survey of Hilltribes in Thailand, 1985–1988*, Office of the Prime Minister, National Statistics Office in Collaboration with the Department of Public Welfare, Bangkok, 1993.

Tribal Research Institute, Chiang Mai University, *A Socio-Cultural Study of the Impact of Social Development programs on Tribal women and children*, Faculty of Social Sciences, Chiang Mai University Press, Chiang Mai, 1985.

Walker, A.R., 'In Mountain and Ulu: A Comparative History of Development Strategies for Ethnic Minority Peoples in Thailand and Malaysia', *Contemporary Southeast Asia*, Vol. 4, No. 4, 1983.

Yu, E.S.H., X. Qiyi, Z. Konglai et al., 'HIV Infection and AIDS in China, 1985–1994', *American Journal of Public Health*, Vol. 86, 1996, pp. 1116–22.

14. Other Genders

Anchalee, Thai Lesbian Network, presentation at the Foreign Correspondents Club of Thailand, Bangkok, September 1995.

Barry, L., *Images Asia*, personal communication, Chiang Mai, 1996.

Beyrer, C., E. Eiumtrakul, D.D. Celentano et al., 'Same-sex behavior, sexually transmitted diseases and HIV risks among young northern Thai men', *AIDS*, Vol. 9, 1995, pp. 171–6.

Herdt, G., *Same Sex, Different Cultures*, Westview, Boulder, 1997.

Jackson, P., *Male Homosexuality in Thailand*, Global Academic Press, New York, 1989.

Kunawarawak, P., P. Parapunya, C. Natpratan, J. Tankayhatt and D. Rojavanavichien, 'KAP and Associated Risk Factor Survey of HIV Infection among Male Commercial Sex Workers in Chiang Mai, December 1992', presentation at the 11th Annual Health Sciences Meeting, Chiang Mai University, 1993.

Lubis, I., J. Master, M. Bambang, A. Papilaya and R.L. Anthony, 'AIDS related attitudes and sexual practices of the Jakarta Waria (male transvestites)', *Southeast Asian Journal of Tropical Medicine and Public Health*, Vol. 25, 1994, pp. 102–6.

Nanda, S., 'Hijras: An Alternative Sex and Gender Role in India', in G. Herdt (ed.), *Third Sex, Third Gender: Beyond Sexual Dimorphism in Culture and History*, Zone Books, New York, 1996.

Nopkesorn, T., M. Sweat, S. Kaensing and T. Teppa, 'Sexual Behaviors for HIV Infection in Young Men in Payao', Research Report No. 6, Program on AIDS, Thai Red Cross Society, 1993.

Patankar, A. (ed.), *The Kamasutra of Vatsyayana*, Hippocrene Books, 1991.

Peltier, A.R., *Pathamamulamuli*, Suriwong Books, Chiang Mai, 1991.
Pradeep, K., M.S. Kumar, Nagarajan and A.J. Hariharan, 'Intervention Development with men who have sex with men in Madras', 10th International Conference on AIDS, Yokohama, Abstract PD0158, 1994.
Rodrigue, Y., *Nat Pwe: Burma's Supernatural Sub-Culture*, Weatherhill, London, 1995.
Sittitrai, W., T. Brown and C. Sakondhavat, 'Levels of HIV risk behavior and AIDS knowledge in Thai men having sex with men', *AIDS Care*, Vol. 5, 1993, pp. 261–71.
Traisupa, A., C. Wongba and D. Taylor, 'AIDS and Prevalence of Antibody to Human Immunodeficiency Virus (HIV) in high risk groups in Thailand', *Genitourinary Medicine*, Vol. 63, 1987, pp. 106–8.

15. Chaai Chuay Chaai

Beyrer, C., A. Artenstein, K. Piyada et al., 'The molecular epidemiology of HIV-1 among male commercial sex workers in northern Thailand', *Journal of AIDS & Human Retrovirology*, Vol. 15, 1997, pp. 304–7.
Kunawararak, P., C. Beyrer, C. Natpratan et al., 'The epidemiology of HIV and syphilis among male commercial sex workers in northern Thailand', *AIDS*, Vol. 9, 1995, pp. 517–21.
de Lind van Wijngaarden, J.W., 'Characteristics, identities, homosexual behavior and condom use among young men in public spaces in urban Chiang Mai, northern Thailand', *NAPAC*, special report, Chiang Mai, 1995.
Varakitphokatorn, S., 'AIDS Risk Among Tourists: A study of Japanese female tourists in Thailand', technical consultation on information regarding population movements and HIV/AIDS, Chulalongkorn University, Bangkok, 1995.

16. Prisons and Prisoners

Amnesty International, 'Myanmar: Conditions in Prisons and Labor Camps', *ASA* 16/22/95, September 1995.
Brien, P.M. and A.J. Beck, *HIV in Prisons, 1994*, US Department of Justice, Bureau of Justice Statistics, Publication NCJ-158020, Washington, D.C., 1996.
Choopanya, K., S. Vanichseni, D.C. Des Jarlais et al., 'Risk factors and HIV seropositivity among injecting drugs users in Bangkok', *AIDS*, Vol. 5, 1991, pp. 1509–13.
Correctional Populations in the United States, 1993, US Department of Justice, Bureau of Justice Statistics, Publication NJ-156241, Washington, D.C., 1995.
Gaiter, J. and L.S. Doll, 'Improving HIV/AIDS Prevention in Prisons is Good Public Health Policy', *American Journal of Public Health*, Vol. 86, 1996, pp. 1201–3.
Mahon, N., 'New York Inmates' HIV Risk Behaviors: The Implications for Prevention Policy and Programs', *American Journal of Public Health*, Vol. 86, 1996, pp. 1211–15.
Win Naing, O., *Cries from Insein*, All Burma Students Democratic Front, Bangkok, 1996.
Wright, N.H., S. Vanichseni, P. Akarasewi, C. Wasi and K. Choopanya, 'Was the

1988 HIV epidemic among Bangkok's injecting drug users a common source outbreak?', *AIDS*, Vol. 8, 1994, pp. 529–32.

17 and 18. The Media and Activists

Anon., 'The Bad Neighbor', *Wall Street Journal*, editorial, November 18, 1996.
New Light of Myanmar, 'The People's Desire' is printed in each daily edition.
Smith, D.K., J.J. Neal, S.D. Homberg et al., 'Unexplained opportunistic infections and CD4+ T-lymphocytopenia without HIV infection', *New England Journal of Medicine*, Vol. 328, 1993, pp. 373–9.
Soto-Ramirez, L.E., B. Renjifo, M.F. McLane et al., 'HIV-1 Langerhans' cell tropism associated with heterosexual transmission of HIV', *Science*, Vol. 271, 1996, pp. 1291–3.

19. Drug Wars and the War on Drugs

Anon., 'Burma's Heroin Deal', editorial, *The Boston Globe*, November 27, 1996.
Bernstein, D. and L. Kean, 'People of the Opiate; Burma's Dictatorship of Drugs', *The Nation*, USA, December 16, 1996, pp. 11–18.
Chee Soon Juan, 'Singapore Sling', *Dateline Interview*, Australian Broadcasting Service, October 12, 1996.
McCoy, A.W., C.B. Reed and C.P. Adams, *The Politics of Heroin in Southeast Asia*, Harper & Row, Singapore, 1972.
Parliament of the Commonwealth of Australia, *A Report on Human Rights and the Lack of Progress Towards Democracy in Burma (Myanmar): The Drug Trade*, Joint Standing Committee of Foreign Affairs, Defense and Trade, Canberra, 1995.
Whitman, W., *Specimen Days*, edited by Mark Van Doren, Viking Press, New York, 1945.

20. Medical Ethics, Human Rights, Asian Values

Cohen, R. and L.S. Wiseberg, *Double Jeopardy – Threat to Life and Human Rights. Discrimination against Persons with AIDS*, Human Rights Internet, Harvard Law School, Cambridge, Mass., 1990.
Farmer, P., *AIDS and Accusation: Haiti and the Geography of Blame*, University of California Press, Berkeley, 1992.
Lintner, B. and H.N. Lintner, 'Blind in Rangoon. AIDS epidemic rages, but the junta says no to NGOs', *Far Eastern Economic Review*, August 1, 1991, p. 21.
MacKinnon, C., 'Crimes of War, Crimes of Peace,' in *On Human Rights, The Oxford Amnesty Lectures 1993*, Basic Books, New York, 1993.
Panos Institute, *The 3rd Epidemic. Repercussions of the Fear of AIDS*, The Panos Institute, London, 1990.

21. Democracy, Empowerment, and Health

Southeast Asian Information Network and EarthRights International, 'Total Denial: A Report on the Yadana Pipeline Project in Burma', SAIN, ERI, Chiang Mai, 1996.

Index

Printed in the United States
17035LVS00001B/42

9 781856 495325